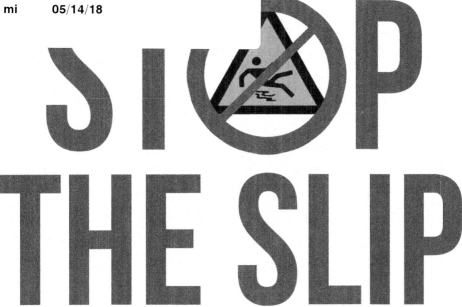

STOP THE SLIP

REDUCING SLIPS, TRIPS AND FALLS
THE #1 CAUSE OF
EMERGENCY ROOM VISITS

THOM DISCH

DEDICATION

This book is dedicated to all of my family members: Kim, Jessi, Alex, Berkeley, Tor, Ashley, Rosie, Josh and Maddox. For the past two years (plus), you've listened to all of my stories and statistics. I appreciate your continuous support, no matter how many family dinners I filled with talk about slips, trips and falls I didn't see a single eye roll or hear a disparaging word. This tremendous support helped me get across the finish line.

Dear reader, this book is also dedicated to all your family members and loved ones. These are the people we spend our lives protecting and keeping safe. If you find just one suggestion or idea that saves a loved one from injury, I've done my job and happily, you have too.

AUTHOR'S NOTE

I've changed the names of the individuals profiled in the sidebars to protect their identity. While all of the sidebars are representative of actual events, some are composites, meaning that I've combined the best lessons from several events to demonstrate how and why a slip, trip, or fall can happen, and then recommend best practices for preventing such events in the future.

For the scientists and technicians in the reading audience: government agencies refer to this class of injury as "slips, trips, and falls," or STF (I use both in this book). These injuries can be a consequence of falling on the same level (this is the most frequent situation) or falling to a lower level, for example, down the stairs or off a ladder. They can also include slipping or tripping without an actual fall; this occurs when a person recovers from a slip, trip, or fall without hitting the ground, but in the process twists or reacts in a way that causes an injury.

Some of the studies and statistics referenced in this book differentiate between these types of occurrences, but many do not. Some even use different groupings, combining the slip or trip without a fall into a "body reaction" injury. Most of the time, this distinction does not affect the conclusion or action plan, so I've merged all of these into the STF category, unless otherwise noted.

Readers who are interested in refining their understanding of the different types of slips, trips, and falls should refer to the original research studies. I've provided detailed footnotes whenever possible.

TABLE OF CONTENTS

───────────────── **SECTION ONE** ─────────────────
Why We Fall   21

—————————————— SECTION TWO ——————————————

Where We Fall   109

—————————————— SECTION THREE ——————————————

The Business Side of Slips, Trips, and Falls   153

──────────────── **SECTION FOUR** ────────────────
Preventing Slips, Trips, and Falls   197

WHY YOU SHOULD READ THIS BOOK

Slip, trip, and fall (STF) injuries are a healthcare crisis in the United States.

Wait, you say, *another* crisis? This must be another attempt to exaggerate a problem just to sell books. If STF injuries really were a major problem, they'd be all over the news. They'd be in the headlines.

You're right. They *should* be in the headlines, but they lack the drama and political intrigue required for headlines today. Furthermore, falls are an everyday occurrence. They happen to everyone, all the time. There's no news there.

The number of people injured and dying from falls is at record numbers and the problem is growing. Using data from 2014, compiled from the Centers for Disease Control database, reveal the true scope of the problem:

- Falls kill three times more people in the United States than firearms and seven times more people than the flu (see Figure 2.3).
- Falls are the number one reason for emergency room visits every year (see Chapter 2, "Why Slips, Trips, and Falls Aren't Taken Seriously" and Figure 2.2).
- Falls cost the US economy over $150 billion per year in medical costs and lost wages (see Chapter 19, "The Cost of Slips, Trips, and Falls").
- Falls are the number one cause of traumatic brain injury, resulting in four times more injuries than sports (see Factoid #2).

- In 2014, falls caused nine million emergency room visits, one million hospitalizations, and thirty thousand deaths (see Chapter 2, "Why Slips, Trips, and Falls Aren't Taken Seriously").
- Falls aren't just a problem for the elderly: 25 percent of fall injuries happen to children and 75 percent happen to people under age 68 (see Chapter 4, "Age and Falls").
- Even though we promote fall safety and prevention for our elderly, the rate at which our elderly die from falls has doubled in the last fifteen years (see Chapter 24, "The ALERT System for Reducing Fall Injuries and Deaths").

You get the picture. The most important message in this book is that you can take some very simple steps to significantly reduce the risk of slips, trips, and falls—and resulting injury or death. Falls don't just happen. They're preceded by a series of events. When you control those preceding events, you reduce the risk of an STF injury (see Section Four, "Preventing Slips, Trips, and Falls").

This book will help you reduce the risk of STF injuries for yourself and the people you care about. As you continue reading, you'll learn about the causes of falls at home and at work. You'll also discover how age, health, occupation, and eyesight can affect the likelihood of a fall. You'll learn that most slips, trips, and falls are avoidable, and that through a process of increasing awareness, training, and implementing an action plan, you can significantly reduce the risk of STF injuries and deaths.

When I started this book, I did what many authors do: I talked about it. I talked to friends, neighbors, vendors, customers, and even casual acquaintances. I became quite the bore, but what I discovered was that *everyone* had a story, and that slips, trips, and falls affect all of us. Each and every person I talked to had a personal experience with a slip, trip, or fall, or knew someone who had been seriously injured or died from a fall. Some had a mother who broke a hip, or a great uncle who suffered a concussion. Others had experienced a fall of their own as a child. Everyone had a connection to this slip, trip, or fall problem.

Although most falls aren't life threatening, they sent more than nine million people to the emergency room in 2014. That's an average of more than one thousand emergency room visits every hour of every day of the year.[1] Falls represent over 30 percent of all emergency department visits. Additionally, injuries caused by slips, trips, and falls aren't limited to the elderly: they're also the number one reason that children (age 16 and under) visit the emergency room every year.[2] And while it's obvious, I want to emphasize these are *emergency room visits* caused by slips and falls. These numbers don't include STF injuries that don't require emergency room attention.

The good news is you can avoid or reduce your chances of becoming an STF statistic. In this book, you'll gain an action plan to avoid slips, trips, and falls for yourself and everyone in your life. I'll provide you with stories, resources, and tips to help you create a personalized safety plan and a checklist to make it easier to eliminate risks.

The book is divided into four sections. Each section starts with some interesting factoids about falls, things I found interesting and hope you'll remember and share as I convert you into a *Stop the Slip* advocate. Each section is independent and can stand alone. Even though Section Four is dedicated specifically to prevention, every section offers additional insights and prevention tips.

Section One: Why We Fall

This section offers some reasons why we don't take slip, trips, and falls—a $150-billion-a-year problem in the United States—more seriously. It explains the mechanics of falling, and describes how age, footwear, weather, medications, alcohol, drugs, pets, and other factors affect the frequency of slips, trips, and falls, and the severity of STF-related injuries.

---

1   Centers for Disease Control and Prevention, "Leading Causes of Nonfatal Injury Reports, 2001–2014," http://webappa.cdc.gov/sasweb/ncipc/nfilead2001.html

2   Ibid.

Section Two: Where We Fall

Most fall injuries happen in or around the home—we're actually much safer from fall injuries when we're at work than when we're away from work. This section identifies the top risk areas and many of the underlying causes that result in accidents. It also offers tips for correcting problems before they cause an injury.

Section Three: The Business Side of Slips, Trips, and Falls

The financial cost of STF injuries are overwhelming, consuming over one percent of GDP in the United States. Slips, trips, and falls are a risk for employees but also impact businesses in other ways. Companies that have customer traffic and higher risk environments have unique challenges. Yet, we are less likely to have an STF injury at work than at home. This section discusses why the work environment is safer and describes the most effective methods businesses are using to reduce STF risks for both customers and employees. It also explores the legal and insurance ramifications of STF injuries, which represent almost 60 percent of all claims processed by insurance companies.

Section Four: Preventing Slips, Trips, and Falls

Falls are a serious health problem for everyone. Our society has focused on emphasizing fall prevention and safety for seniors because they are the most at risk for STF injuries or worse. The results of those prevention programs are disappointing. This section presents the ALERT System for reducing fall injuries, providing a simple, yet actionable set of steps that will help you reduce the risk for yourself and the people you care about. It concludes with checklists and safety audits you can use to identify and eliminate fall risks in every room of your home and workplace.

The first and most important step in preventing slips, trips, and falls is to increase awareness of the problem. By taking the actions outlined in this book, you can make the world a safer place and protect the people you know and love from unnecessary pain and suffering.

Many people have shared the intimate details of their pain and suffering to help us learn how to be safer. Many others have studied the issue and compiled great statistical analyses to highlight the extent of this problem. I hope that I've been able combine their stories and research into an interesting resource, so that we can begin a broader conversation about reducing these injuries. It all begins with you and then you telling two people—and then them telling two people.

In conjunction with this book, you can find useful digital tools, new information, breaking stories, and evolving trends and statistics in the world of slips, trips, and falls at stoptheslip.com.

I hope you enjoy this book.
Thom Disch

CHAPTER 1

ANNE AND JOHN

Take a moment and think back to the last time you went on vacation. Better yet, think about your last great vacation—the one that you spent months planning and anticipating. Place yourself back into that time when you were getting ready to leave. Remember the excitement as you finished packing? Remember all the last-minute things you had to do before you left? This is the moment where we meet Anne and John.

Anne and John were married almost ten years ago. Right after their wedding they bought their perfect home. They took many small vacations and long weekend trips. But, as is true for many two-income couples, planning for a big vacation came with its own set of challenges. When Anne's workload was light, John was in the middle of a crisis, and vice versa. In celebration of their ten-year anniversary they planned a three-week trip across Europe. All the details were worked out and they were ready to go.

The morning they planned on leaving, John opened the front door. He normally used the door through the garage, but he'd already pulled the car around. Suitcases in hand, he stepped out onto the porch and started to descend the stairs. The air was just a bit nippy and the stairs still had a coating of morning dew on them. His leather-soled shoes slipped. As he struggled to regain his balance and hold onto the suitcases, his foot slipped forward, and John fell backward.

Anne heard John cry out and looked up in time to see him and the suitcases fall to the steps. When he fell, John hit the back of his head on the edge of the top porch step, making a sound that Anne described as "sickening." She ran to his side and had time to tell him, "It's going to be okay," before he lost consciousness. She took off her sweater, rolled it up, and placed it under his head. She told him not to move and ran back into the house to call an ambulance.

John was taken to the intensive care unit with a traumatic brain injury. Anne believed they had done everything right, and she never stopped questioning why everything had all gone wrong. One slip and life as they each knew it ended. No future, no travel, nothing.

Anne and John were like many of us. They had planned for every aspect of their trip, from insurance, airfare, hotels, and meals to spare medications to carry with them. They even discussed what they would do if one of them were injured in a foreign country. What they never thought about was how slippery the front porch might be the morning they were set to leave.

Sadly, this isn't an isolated type of incident. But by changing the way we think, we can avoid most slips, trips, and falls. The goal is to implement an action plan that will help reduce your risk.

No one thinks a fall will happen to them. It's always someone else. We watch YouTube videos and TV shows about how funny people look when they fall and we think: "What a klutz! I'm glad I'm not that guy!" or "That poor girl! I'm just glad it wasn't me." And then we go back to our daily lives and forget all about it. As of right now, make a conscious effort to realize that *we are those people.* Every person who is injured by a fall is surprised by that fall. This book will teach you how to identify and avoid high-risk situations and to ultimately *Stop the Slip.*

Here are three actions that could have prevented John's fall, or lessened its severity:

- Anne and John lived in this house for many years. They were certainly aware that their front porch stairs could be slippery. They most likely slipped on this porch at one time or another but avoided serious injury at that time. It's common to recognize a slip-and-fall hazard but not take action to prevent a future fall injury. See Chapter 11, "Stairs and Handrails," for several options for fixing slippery steps.
- John could have made a better footwear choice. He was wearing shoes that were comfortable and fashionable. The problem was that many of

these high-end shoes have leather soles, which are flat and notoriously slippery. Shoes designed with a rubberized, nonslip sole are much safer and minimize the risk of falling. Do you prioritize fashion over safety when selecting a pair of shoes? See Chapter 5, "Footwear," for more on this subject.

- John was carrying two suitcases as he walked out to the car. This meant that he had both hands full, so he couldn't hold the handrail to steady himself after he slipped. And he couldn't use his hands to break his fall or protect his head. See Chapter 11, "Stairs and Handrails," for more on this subject.

After two years of researching this book, I'm convinced: **everyone has a slip, trip, and fall story**. The purpose of sharing this story is to increase your awareness of the problem, to reduce or eliminate your embarrassment over falling (so you won't hide from the problem), and to provide a platform for learning prevention techniques that will help you avoid painful and costly fall injuries.

SECTION ONE

Why We Fall

Ask *why* five times. I was taught in journalism class that to get to the root of a problem you need to ask *why* five times. In this section, we'll explore the question of why we fall. We'll ask and discuss why from several different perspectives. And we'll discuss the four primary reasons that falls—the number one reason for emergency room visits in the United States—are a growing problem and why we as a society aren't taking them seriously:

- Falls are seen as humorous.
- Falls aren't considered dangerous.
- We have an optimism bias.
- We lack fall-prevention advocates.

We'll discuss what causes an actual fall and the resulting injuries. We'll discuss how age affects us and our personal fall risk. Today, the elderly are the primary focus of research on falls. But we actually fall more when we're younger (see Chapter 4, "Age and Falls"). We'll dig into the statistics that show why everyone is at risk for a slip, trip, and fall injury. We'll explore why the elderly are the focus of fall prevention programs even though 75 percent of the fall injuries that require a trip to the emergency room are for falls suffered by individuals under the age of 68. (Don't worry: most of the numbers are presented as charts and graphs that make them easier to understand.)

We'll finish this section with a look at the decisions we make, like what shoes to wear, that contribute to our personal slip, trip, and fall risk. And we'll examine the environmental factors that contribute to fall risk. For example, even though we intuitively know that ice and snow increase our risk for fall injuries, the numbers show that winter isn't when most fall deaths occur. The complex nature of falls indicate that there's more than one solution to the problem.

This section will increase your awareness of the fall crisis in the United States; this knowledge is the first step in developing your personal fall prevention system, which we'll discuss in the final section of the book.

Section One Factoids

As I was writing this book, I discovered that the best way to catch people's interest was to tell them a surprising fact about slip, trip, and fall (STF) injuries. These factoids became a hit around the office and were a quick way to create interest in the STF topic. They also gave the person I was talking with a conversation starter that they could share with their friends and family to convey the seriousness of STFs. I've included five surprising factoids about STFs at the start of each section of the book. I've also made it easy to share them: you can download a printer-friendly, color version of all twenty factoids at stoptheslip.com/factoids. You can print them on a standard US letter-size sheet of paper and post them on your company bulletin board, outside your cubicle or office, or even on your refrigerator at home. Because there are twenty of them you can change them once a week and keep the message fresh.

Got additional factoids you'd like to share? E-mail them to me at Thom@stoptheslip.com and include your source so I can verify the information. I'll be sure to credit you for any factoids that you contribute.

Falls were the number one cause of emergency room visits in 2014

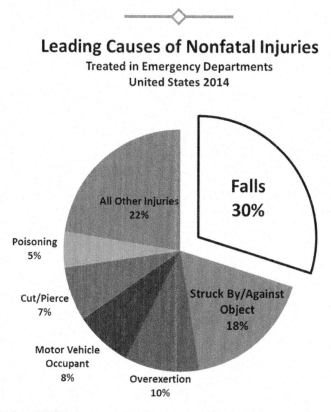

Leading Causes of Nonfatal Injuries
Treated in Emergency Departments
United States 2014

Falls
30%

All Other Injuries
22%

Poisoning
5%

Cut/Pierce
7%

Motor Vehicle
Occupant
8%

Overexertion
10%

Struck By/Against
Object
18%

Data Source: NEISS All Injury Program operated by the Consumer Product Safety Commission (CPSC).
National Center for Injury Prevention and Control, CDC using WISQARS™. Data Extracted September 1, 2016.

- Falls have been the number one cause of ER visits for the past 15 years
- Falls have causes over 100 million ER visits since 2001
- Falls cause almost 4 times more ER visits than motor vehicles.

Falls are the leading cause of traumatic brain injury (TBI)

—◇—

Causes of Traumatic Brain Injury

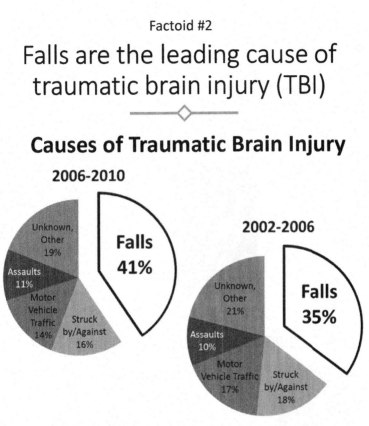

2006-2010

Unknown, Other 19%
Assaults 11%
Motor Vehicle Traffic 14%
Struck by/Against 16%
Falls 41%

2002-2006

Unknown, Other 21%
Assaults 10%
Motor Vehicle Traffic 17%
Struck by/Against 18%
Falls 35%

Data Source: Studies by Centers for Disease Control; www.cdc.gov/traumaticbraininjury/get_the_facts.html; and www.cdc.gov/traumaticbraininjury/pdf/BlueBook_factsheet-a.pdf

- Falls cause four times more TBIs than sports.
- Falls cause three times more TBIs than motor vehicle traffic.
- Falls as a cause of TBI have gotten progressively worse in recent years.

Factoid #3

Falls Cause More Injuries and Deaths Than Gun Violence

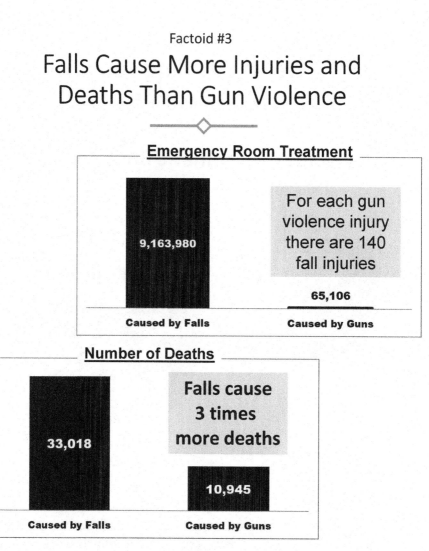

Emergency Room Treatment

9,163,980

For each gun violence injury there are 140 fall injuries

65,106

Caused by Falls   **Caused by Guns**

Number of Deaths

33,018

Falls cause 3 times more deaths

10,945

Caused by Falls   **Caused by Guns**

Data Source: NEISS All Injury Program operated by the Consumer Product Safety Commission (CPSC).
National Center for Injury Prevention and Control, CDC using WISQARS™. Data Extracted September 1, 2016.

Many lives could be saved and injuries avoided if we invested as much time and money in fall prevention campaigns as we do in gun control advocacy.

Factoid #4

Falls are causing more deaths than ever before

◇

Percentage of All Deaths Caused by Falls
In the United States

1.40%	
1.20%	1.22%
1.00%	1.17%
	1.13%
	1.09%
	1.05%
	1.02%
	0.97%
	0.93%
0.80%	0.86%
	0.80%
	0.78%
	0.70%
	0.67%
0.60%	0.62%
	0.55% 0.55%
0.40%	
0.20%	
0.00%	

1999 2000 2001 2002 2003 2004 2005 2006 2007 2008 2009 2010 2011 2012 2013 2014

Calculations and Chart Design: Thom Disch for "Stop The Slip"
Data Source: NEISS All Injury Program operated by the Consumer Product Safety Commission (CPSC).
National Center for Injury Prevention and Control, CDC using WISQARS™.

Falls have grown from causing 0.55% of all deaths in 1999 to causing 1.22% of all deaths in 2014.

This is an increase of over 120% during the last 15 years.

Falls are now the 14th leading cause of death in the US.

Factoid #5

Serious fall injuries happen to everyone regardless of age

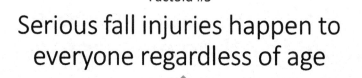

Fall Injuries - Fall Hospitalizations - Fall Deaths
By Age Group in 2013

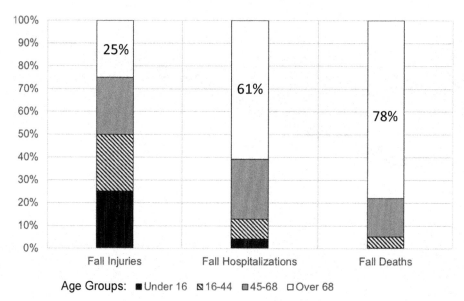

Data Source: NEISS All Injury Program operated by the Consumer Product Safety Commission (CPSC).
National Center for Injury Prevention and Control, CDC using WISQARS™. [Data extracted on September 1, 2015]

Fall Injuries are injuries that result in an emergency room visit

- 25% of fall injuries happen to each of these age groups: Under 16; 16 to 44; 45 to 68; and over 68 years of age.
- Youth do not have as many serious consequences from falls.
- While only 25% of fall injuries happen to people over 68, they result in 61% of the hospitalizations and 78% of the deaths caused by falls.

CHAPTER 2

WHY SLIPS, TRIPS, AND FALLS AREN'T TAKEN SERIOUSLY

Fall injuries are at a crisis level in The United States. It's one of the largest chronic health problems we face today. And the problem is getting worse. Yet falls and their prevention aren't mainstream topics of conversation. While researching this book, I talked with thousands of people, and when I brought up the subject, everyone had a personal experience with a slip, trip, and fall tragedy. So, if this is a serious problem that touches all of us, why aren't we taking action to reduce the number of injuries and deaths from falls?

Before we answer that question, let's look at the facts:

Falls are consistently the number one reason people go to the emergency room. In 2014, falls caused 9.2 million emergency room visits, representing 30 percent of all emergency room visits (Figure 2.1).[3] They've been the number one reason people go to the emergency room for as long as the Centers for Disease Control and Prevention (CDC) have had an online database. In fact,

---

3   National Center for Injury Prevention and Control, Centers for Disease Control and Prevention, We-b-Based Injury Statistics Query and Reporting System (WISQARS). www.cdc.gov/ncipc/wisqars.

emergency room visits from falls exceed the number of emergency room visits from auto accidents by a factor of three.

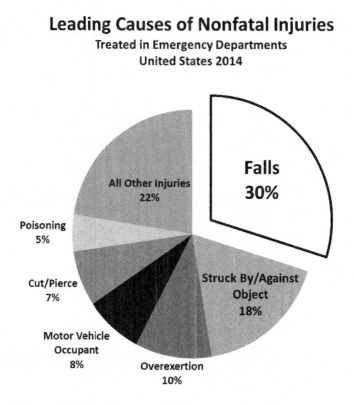

Leading Causes of Nonfatal Injuries
Treated in Emergency Departments
United States 2014

Falls
30%

All Other Injuries
22%

Poisoning
5%

Cut/Pierce
7%

Motor Vehicle
Occupant
8%

Overexertion
10%

Struck By/Against
Object
18%

Data Source: NEISS All Injury Program operated by the Consumer Product Safety Commission (CPSC). National Center for Injury Prevention and Control, CDC using WISQARS™.

FIGURE 2.1 Leading causes of nonfatal injuries treated in emergency rooms in the United States, 2014

Fall injuries have grown from 26 percent of all emergency room treated injuries in 2001 to 30 percent in 2014 (Figure 2.2). This was happening as the other major causes of emergency room visits have declined.[4] The results of STF emergency room visits included over one million hospitalizations.[5]

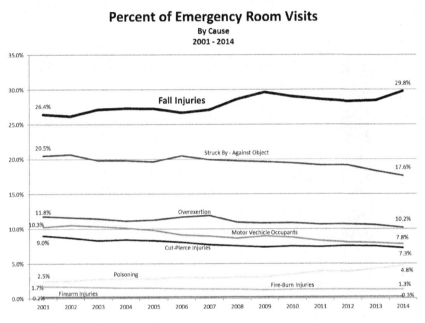

Chart Design: Thom Disch for *Stop The Slip*
Data Source: NEISS All Injury Program operated by the Consumer Product Safety Commission (CPSC). National Center for Injury Prevention and Control, CDC using WISQARS™.

FIGURE 2.2 Percentage of emergency room visits by cause, 2001–2014

4   Ibid.
5   Ibid.

In 2014, falls were the fourteenth leading cause of death in the United States, resulting in 31,959 fatalities (Figure 2.3).[6] By comparison, falls killed three times more people than firearm homicides and seven times more people than the flu.

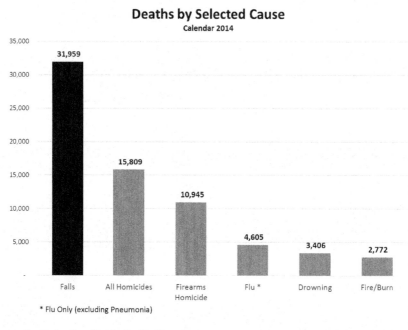

Deaths by Selected Cause
Calendar 2014

* Flu Only (excluding Pneumonia)

Chart Design: Thom Disch for *Stop The Slip*
Data Sources: NEISS All Injury Program operated by the Consumer Product Safety Commission (CPSC).
National Center for Injury Prevention and Control, CDC using WISQARS™ and National Vital Statistics Reports

FIGURE 2.3 Deaths by selected cause, 2014

For further emphasis, the percentage of deaths caused by falls is growing at a rapid pace. In 1999, falls caused 0.55 percent of all deaths in the United States (Figure 2.4). By 2014, that percentage more than doubled to 1.22 percent.

---

6   Ibid. (For a table of the top fifteen causes of death in the United States, go to http://stoptheslip.com/book/topcausesofdeath.)

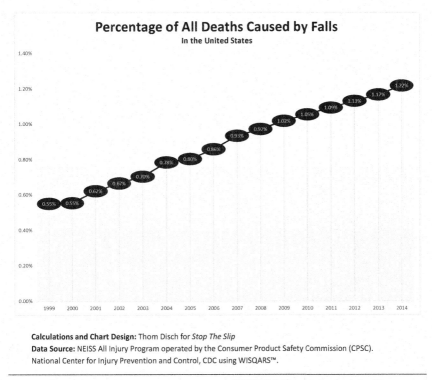

Calculations and Chart Design: Thom Disch for *Stop The Slip*
Data Source: NEISS All Injury Program operated by the Consumer Product Safety Commission (CPSC). National Center for Injury Prevention and Control, CDC using WISQARS™.

FIGURE 2.4 Percentage of deaths caused by falls in the United States

The facts are undeniable: STF injuries are a chronic problem in the United States. The data comes straight from the CDC. Most safety and healthcare professionals aren't surprised by this information; they're faced with the problem every day at work. So why isn't fall prevention at the top of our action list? Why isn't it headline news every day? The simple answer is perception. We don't perceive fall injuries as a serious problem. The more complex answer shows us four factors that have numbed us to the danger of STF injuries:

- Falls are seen as humorous.
- Falls aren't considered dangerous.
- We have an optimism bias.

• We lack fall-prevention advocates.

Falls are seen as humorous

What do Dick Van Dyke, Chevy Chase, and *America's Funniest Home Videos* have in common? They represent just a few examples of how falls have been used as humor on television. In the 1960s, at the start of every episode of the *Dick Van Dyke Show*, Rob Petrie either tripped over or dodged an ottoman in the center of his living room. In the 1970s, Chevy Chase began his iconic TV and film career on *Saturday Night Live* doing pratfalls of President Gerald Ford (this actually resulted in a back injury for Mr. Chase, with chronic back pain and addiction to painkillers).[7] Today, YouTube is flooded with videos of everyday people hilariously surviving slips, trips, and falls.

Of course, falls as humor didn't start with the television era; they've been considered entertaining since the days of ancient Egypt and are an integral part of vaudeville and slapstick comedy.[8] And there's actually a psychological reward to watching the misfortune of others. (If you want to know more about this, look up the word *schadenfreude*.) If you're one of those people who find slip, trip, and fall videos funny, don't feel too guilty; psychologists who've researched this topic say that most everyone experiences some form of this.[9]

When watching someone slip, trip, and fall, the mind goes through a series of thoughts, perhaps something like this: mental cringe; that must have hurt; glad it's not me; wow, that guy looks pretty silly; it's kind of funny; chuckle, giggle, chuckle; look around to make sure no one saw your amusement at someone else's pain. Unfortunately, the fact that our brains are programmed to find falls humorous diminishes the seriousness of the slip, trip, and fall problem and lessens our perception of the risks and damage caused by falls.

---

7   UPI, "Chevy Chase Being Treated For Addiction to Painkillers," The New York Times, October 12, 1986, http://www.nytimes.com/1986/10/12/us/chevy-chase-being-treated-for-addiction-to-painkillers.html.

8   Josh Sanburn, "A Brief History of Slapstick Humor," *Time*, October 18, 2010, http://content.time.com/time/arts/article/0,8599,2025795,00.html.

9   Jeanna Bryner, "Schadenfreude Explained: Why We Secretly Smile When Others Fail," *Live Science*, December 9, 2011, http://www.livescience.com/17398-schadenfreude-affirmation.html.

Falls aren't considered dangerous

But wait, you say: We don't laugh at gunshot victims or auto accidents. Why are falls different? This is partly related to the relative violence and severity of each of these events. You can immediately see this when you mentally replay at the moment of impact for each event.

We can quantify this by comparing the fatality rate for each event. To calculate a fatality rate, divide the number of people who died from an event by the number of people injured by that event. The higher the fatality rate, the more violent/severe the event. Figure 2.5 shows the fatality rates for several events. The more violent the event the more seriously the event is treated.

Fatality Rate
Calendar 2013

Event	Fatality Rate	
Firearm Assault	15.7994%	More Violent/Severe
Poisoning	3.5486%	
Motor Vehicles	0.8621%	
Fire/Burns	0.7119%	
Falls	0.3432%	
Struck By/Against	0.0170%	
Overexertion	0.0004%	Less Violent/Severe

Calculations: The percentage of people receiving medical attention that die as a result of their injuries by Thom Disch for *Stop The Slip*
Data Source: NEISS All Injury Program operated by the Consumer Product Safety Commission (CPSC). National Center for Injury Prevention and Control, CDC using WISQARS™.

FIGURE 2.5 Fatality rate

For example, the firearm assault fatality rate is 15.8 percent, meaning that one out of every six gunshot victims dies from those injuries. For motor vehicle accident victims, it's 0.86 percent; one out of every 116 people receiving medical attention dies. For falls, 0.34 percent of the people receiving medical attention die, which translates into one person dying for every 291 receiving medical attention. Being struck by or against an object is even less violent and severe than a fall. And if you've ever watched the *Three Stooges* or other variations of slapstick comedy, you'd have to agree that being struck by or against an object could belong in the humor category.

We can also factor in the personal familiarity we all have with slips, trips, and falls. Think back over the last few weeks—you'll most likely remember a slip, trip, or fall. I don't mean a catastrophic event, but rather a little slip in the kitchen from water that splashed out of the sink or a little stumble on an uneven sidewalk. Such a minor occurrence didn't result in an injury and (if no one was watching) you probably forgot about it quickly. But it *did* leave an imprint on your subconscious. Since we experience many slips, trips, and falls that don't result in an injury, those events convince us that slips, trips, and falls aren't dangerous.

Let's try an experiment. Consider the two signs shown in Figure 2.6, both of which you've probably seen in the past couple of weeks:

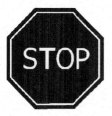 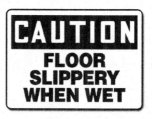

FIGURE 2.6 Stop and caution signs

When you come to the Stop sign, unless you're irresponsible and reckless, you're going to stop, or at least slow down. When you come to the Caution sign, do you have a similar reaction? Probably not. Why? Because if you ignore the Stop sign, you believe really bad things will happen (auto accident or traffic ticket). We need to realize that ignoring the Caution sign can certainly result in a serious accident and injury.

Our experience with slips, trips, and falls has shown us that we can typically avoid serious injury until the right set of circumstances occurs. (As we age, the likelihood that we'll have a serious injury from a slip, trip, or fall increases, and that increases our caution relating to fall risks, but we'll talk more about that later.) The statistics at the beginning of this chapter make a case for changing our perception about STF risk.

The nature of our human programming supports this misperception and leads us to the next contribution factor: optimism bias.

Sean

Sean is sledding with a group of friends on a snowy hill. As is often the case with teenagers, they've been looking for ways to up the ante, now that the simple act of rocketing down a hill on a sled has started to feel routine. Sean has a bright idea.

"Watch this!" he says. He positions a sled at the peak of the hill and steps back, gauging the distance. A friend asks what he's doing. "I'm gonna run, jump on it, land standing up, and ride it down like a snowboard!" They egg him on, eager to see the result. After all, none of them have ever been seriously hurt from a fall, and they're young, and the ground is covered with snow, and what's the worst that could happen?

Sean gets a running start, jumps, lands, and of course, the sled shoots out from under him. The back of his head hits the ground first. He's lucky. The snow saves him from worse damage. But the fact that he did not get seriously hurt makes him feel like he's as invincible as ever.

Sound familiar? Probably, if you were ever a kid.

We have an optimism bias

People are optimistic by nature. The Prudential Insurance Company surveyed more than 2,400 people, asking them to share important events that happened to them in the past and events that might happen to them in the future. If someone is realistic, you would expect the mix of good to bad events in their past to be same as they predict in their future. If they're pessimistic, the future would have more bad events. If they're optimistic, the future would have more good events. When researchers analyzed the mix of good and bad events, they discovered that people went from a historical 40 percent bad to a future of only 16 percent bad (Figure 2.7). That's a dramatic drop, indicating that people don't expect negative things to happen in their future.[10]

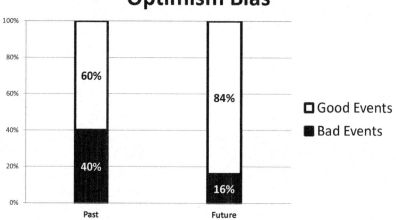

Data Source: The Prudential Insurance Company; The Prudential Magnets Experiment; Survey of 2400 people asked to list events in their past and events in their future; February 2015

FIGURE 2.7 Optimism bias

---

10   Prudential Financial, Inc., "It Won't Happen to Me: Exploring Our Tendency to Be Overly Optimistic and How It Affects Our Long-Term Financial Plans," http://www.bringyourchallenges.com/it-wont-happen-to-me#magnets.

This optimism bias is one of the factors that increase our risk of falling.[11] It encouraged Sean to use his sled as a snowboard and it causes us to calculate risks in a way that overestimates the chances of experiencing positive events while underestimating the chances of encountering negative events.[12] We generally act as if things will go well and not end in calamity. The resulting overzealous attitude of "it won't happen to me" can lead to not paying attention to our environment, heeding warning signs, or eliminating known STF hazards. In the end, we don't take common sense precautions to prevent slips, trips, and falls.

Optimism bias is also more prevalent in people over age 60. One reason for this has been shown by behavioral economist Andrew Oswald. Oswald's research shows that we start life full of happiness and optimism, which diminishes significantly during middle age, and then returns as we advance into our older years.[13] His conclusion: older people are likely to be more satisfied and happier than those who are middle-aged. This satisfaction makes us less cautious and more willing to take a risk. Oswald's research is consistent with why STF accidents increase as we get older. Just to be clear, I'm not saying that it is a primary cause of falls in the elderly but it may be a contributing factor. We'll discuss slips, trips, and falls associated with aging in a later section.

---

11 Tali Sharot, "The Optimism Bias," *Current Biology* 21, no. 23 (2011): R941–R945, doi: 10.1016/j. cub.2011.10.030.

12 Adam Dachis, "Your Optimism Bias: One of the Best and Worst Tricks Your Brain Plays on You," *Life Hacker*, May 18, 2012, http://lifehacker.com/5911556/ your-optimism-bias-the-best-and-worst-thing-your-brain-can-do-for-you.

13 Tali Sharot, "Optimism Bias: Why the Young and the Old Tend to Look on the Bright Side," *Washington Post*, December 31, 2012, https://www.washingtonpost.com/national/health-science/ optimism-bias-why-the-young-and-the-old-tend-to-look-on-the-bright-side/2012/12/28/ac4147de-37f8-11e2-a263-f0ebffed2f15_story.html.

We lack fall-prevention advocates

The fall data for people of working age (18 to 65) shows that only 6 percent of injuries and 16 percent of deaths occur at work (see Figure 2.8).[14] After adjusting for time spent sleeping, labor force participation, and driving time, people between the ages of 18 and 65 spend approximately 27 percent of their time at work.[15] That's quite a disparity. All things being equal, if we spend 27 percent of our time at work, we would expect that 27 percent of fall injuries and deaths would occur at work. However, the data clearly shows that we're much safer *at* work than *away* from work. (See Chapter 21, "Types of Work Environments," for more details.)

---

14 Centers for Disease Control and Prevention, Injury Prevention and Control: Data and Statistics, https://www.cdc.gov/injury/wisqars/index.html, and Bureau of Labor Statistics, Injuries, Illnesses and Fatalities Databases, http://www.bls.gov/iif/data.htm.

15 For those who are interested here's how the math works: There are 168 hours in a week; During an average week we spend 8 hours driving and 48 hours sleeping, times when it is difficult to fall; Removing that time we are left with 112 hours of at risk fall-time per week; The average working person spends an average of 47 hours at work, but not everyone works, the labor force participation rate is approximately 64%, so 47 hours times 64% means that the general population spends, on average, 30 hours per week at work; Dividing this 30 hours of work-time by the potential fall-time of 112 hours gives us 26.8%. If fall injuries happen at the same rate when we are at work and when we are not at work we would expect that 26.8% of fall injuries to happen at work.

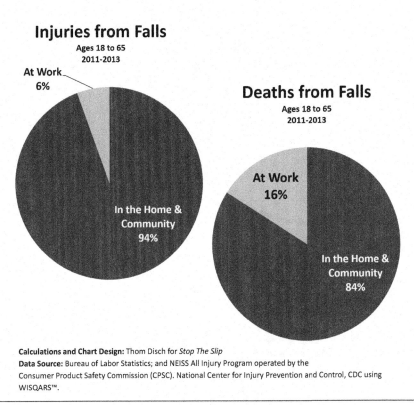

Injuries from Falls
Ages 18 to 65
2011-2013

At Work
6%

In the Home &
Community
94%

Deaths from Falls
Ages 18 to 65
2011-2013

At Work
16%

In the Home &
Community
84%

Calculations and Chart Design: Thom Disch for *Stop The Slip*
Data Source: Bureau of Labor Statistics; and NEISS All Injury Program operated by the
Consumer Product Safety Commission (CPSC). National Center for Injury Prevention and Control, CDC using
WISQARS™.

FIGURE 2.8 Injuries and deaths from
falls, ages 18 to 65, 2011–2013

From 1999 to 2014, the number of deaths caused by motor vehicle accidents dropped 18 percent (from 41,000 in 1999 to 34,000 in 2014), while the total number of miles driven grew by 10 percent and the number of drivers grew by 14 percent (Figure 2.9). Conversely, the number of deaths caused by falls has risen a dramatic 137 percent (13,000 in 1999 to 33,000 in 2014), while the total population has grown by only 14 percent.[16]

16 Centers for Disease Control and Prevention, Injury Prevention and Control: Data and Statistics, https://www.cdc.gov/injury/wisqars/index.html.

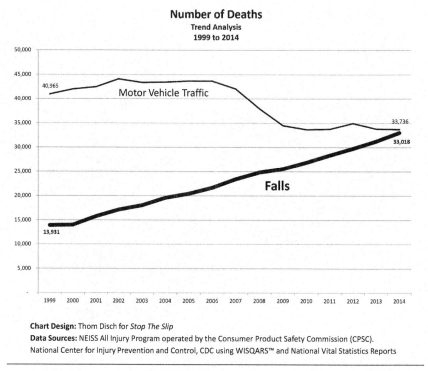

Number of Deaths
Trend Analysis
1999 to 2014

Chart Design: Thom Disch for *Stop The Slip*
Data Sources: NEISS All Injury Program operated by the Consumer Product Safety Commission (CPSC).
National Center for Injury Prevention and Control, CDC using WISQARS™ and National Vital Statistics Reports

FIGURE 2.9 Number of deaths, trend analysis, 1999–2014

Injuries and deaths caused by falls on the job are dramatically lower than we might expect. The number of drivers and miles driven has grown, yet deaths and injuries from motor vehicle accidents have declined substantially. Why do these injury trends contradict expectations? We can thank advocacy groups and governmental agencies whose explicit mission is raising awareness of the problem and reducing the risks of harm from a specific cause.

The workplace has the Occupational Safety and Health Administration (OSHA) and the focused support of every insurance agency that provides workers' compensation insurance. The result is that every business has dedicated resources to make the workplace safer. There are jobs and careers dedicated to protecting employees and reducing the number of fall injuries.

The roadways have many advocates. The National Highway Traffic Safety Administration (NHTSA) and Mothers Against Drunk Driving (MADD) are two of the more notable organizations dedicated to reducing accidents and deaths related to motor vehicles.

While several organizations discuss the importance of fall prevention, there are no high-profile, dedicated advocacy groups working to reduce injuries from falls in our everyday lives. Huge amounts of money are dedicated to meeting OSHA and NHTSA guidelines. Looking at what has been accomplished in making all of us safer at work and on the roads proves that we can reduce the number of fall injuries and deaths with the right amount of effort and attention. You'll learn more about this in Section Four, "Preventing Slips, Trips, and Falls."

Standards and Guidelines for STF Prevention

In researching this book, I looked for guidelines and standards that could be used to help prevent slips, trips, and falls. What I found was interesting. There are more standards created for using fall protection equipment than for addressing falls on the same level. Because of the serious consequences of a fall from a height that makes some sense, but the lack of standards relating to falls on the same level is surprising.

OSHA recognizes STFs as a serious problem, stating: "Slips, trips, and falls constitute the majority of general industry accidents. They cause 15% of all accidental deaths, and are second only to motor vehicles as a cause of fatalities."[17] OSHA does take fall injuries very seriously and they have a section dedicated to standards for "Walking-Working Surfaces," however this section focuses on falls from a height rather than on falls on the same level. The only mention of same-level falls in this standard is as follows:

---

17   Occupational Safety and Health Administration, Safety and Health Topics: Walking/Working Surfaces, https://www.osha.gov/SLTC/walkingworkingsurfaces/.

1910 Subpart D: Walking-Working Surfaces, Standard 22 General requirements

1910.22(a) Housekeeping. (1) All places of employment, passageways, storerooms, and service rooms shall be kept clean and orderly and in a sanitary condition.

(2) The floor of every workroom shall be maintained in a clean and, so far as possible, a dry condition. Where wet processes are used, drainage shall be maintained, and false floors, platforms, mats, or other dry standing places should be provided where practicable.

(3) To facilitate cleaning, every floor, working place, and passageway shall be kept free from protruding nails, splinters, holes, or loose boards.

The Americans with Disabilities Act (ADA) states that floor surfaces must be slip resistant, but it provides no standard for how to measure slip resistance. It does address changes in elevation, which might represent a tripping hazard, indicating that up to one-quarter inch change in elevation is acceptable without modification and up to one-half inch change in elevation is acceptable if the height above one-quarter inch is cut with a slope.[18] Note that these standards were primarily created to support the disabled community and not the general public.

The American National Standards Institute (ANSI), a nonprofit organization that administers and coordinates the US voluntary standards, has worked with the National Floor Safety Institute (NFSI) to create the most complete same-level fall prevention standards:

- ANSI/NFSI B101.0 Walkway Surface Auditing Procedure for the Measurement of Walkway Slip Resistance
- ANSI/NFSI B101.1 Test Method for Measuring Wet Static Coefficient of Friction of Common Hard-Surface Floor Materials

---

18   United States Access Board, Chapter 3: Floor and Ground Surfaces, www.access-board.gov/guidelines-and-standards/buildings-and-sites/about-the-ada-standards/guide-to-the-ada-standards/chapter-3-floor-and-ground-surfaces#303

- ANSI/NFSI B101.3 Test Method for Measuring Wet Dynamic Coefficient of Friction of Common Hard-Surface Floor Materials (Including Action and Limit Thresholds for the Suitable Assessment of the Measured Values)
- ANSI/NFSI B101.5 Standard Guide for Uniform Labeling Method for Identifying the Wet Static Coefficient of Friction (Traction) of Floor Coverings, Floor Coverings with Coatings, and Treated Floor Coverings
- ANSI/NFSI B101.6 Standard Guide for Commercial Entrance Matting in Reducing Slips, Trips, and Falls

The detailed standards can be found at either the ANSI or the NFSI websites.[19]

---

19   ANSI: http://webstore.ansi.org/ and then search for ANSI/NFSI B101
     NFSI: https://nfsi.org/ansinfsi-standards/standards/

CHAPTER 3

SLIPS, TRIPS, AND FALLS: THE INSIDE STORY

According to the Centers for Disease Control and Prevention (CDC), STF injuries cost the US economy over $172 billion in 2013.[20] That cost includes the medical and lifetime work-loss costs from fall injuries. Slips, trips, and falls are a big problem in the United States and around the world. To stop these injuries, we need to better understand the problem. Fortunately for us, thousands of studies have looked at the STF problem. Fortunately for you, you don't have to sort through the data because I've done that and tried to relate it to everyday life.

In the United States, there are two primary databases that capture information on STF-related injuries and deaths. One is managed by the CDC; the other is managed by the Bureau of Labor Statistics (BLS). The CDC's Web-Based Injury Statistics Query and Reporting System (WISQARS) is an interactive database that provides US injury data including fatal and nonfatal

---

20 Curtis Florence, et al., "Estimated Lifetime Medical and Work-Loss Costs of Emergency Department–Treated Nonfatal Injuries—United States, 2013," *Morbidity and Mortality Weekly Report* 64, no. 38: 1078–1082, http://www.cdc.gov/mmwr/preview/mmwrhtml/mm6438a5.htm?s_cid=mm6438a5_w.

injury, violent death, and cost of injury data from a variety of trusted sources.[21] The CDC compiles data related to daily living and the general population. The BLS's Injuries, Illnesses, and Fatalities (IIF) program provides annual information on the rate and number of work-related injuries, illnesses, and fatal injuries, and how these statistics vary by incident, industry, geography, occupation, and other characteristics.[22] The BLS data focuses on events that occur at work or are related to work.

In preparing stories and prevention advice for the STF problem, I pulled data from these two databases or from studies that were compiled by professional researchers. The sources of the data are documented in the footnotes, so you can take a deeper look.[23]

A fall occurs when you lose your balance and your body hits the ground or something on the way down. This impact is typically what causes an injury or worse. The BLS tracks the cause of injuries that result in time off from work (Figure 3.1). Looking specifically at injuries from slips, trips, and falls, they fall into three major classifications: falls on the same level (63 percent), falls from elevation (19 percent), and slips or trips without a fall (16 percent). I was surprised by the number of injuries from slips and trips without a fall, which cause you to pull a muscle or tweak something. One of my more cynical editors suggested that the percentage of these injuries (16 percent) was artificially high because some workers claim a fake injury to get paid time off from the worker's compensation insurance program. There's no statistical evidence to support this contention. I bring it up only because the topic sparked an interesting but unresolvable debate. I'll leave this issue to your own personal level of cynicism.

---

21   Centers for Disease Control and Prevention, Injury Prevention and Control: Data and Statistics, http://www.cdc.gov/injury/wisqars/facts.html.

22   United States Department of Labor, Bureau of Labor Statistics, http://www.bls.gov/iif/.

23   If you have a different interpretation of the data or a different perspective, I invite you to e-mail me at Thom@stoptheslip.com. I look forward to hearing about your experiences and to working together to prevent STF injuries.

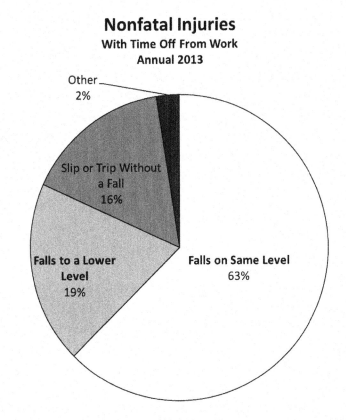

Nonfatal Injuries
With Time Off From Work
Annual 2013

Data Source: U.S. Department of Labor, Bureau of Labor Statistics. Injuries, Illnesses and Fatalities Database.

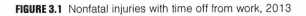

FIGURE 3.1 Nonfatal injuries with time off from work, 2013

Keep in mind that this is only for work-related injuries. The CDC database doesn't track this level of detail, so we don't know if this same causation pattern for injuries occurs away from the workplace.

Falls in the business world

The Centers for Disease Control (CDC) treats all fall injuries the same. Whether you fall in the bathtub or fall off a ladder the CDC classifies this as a fall injury (or a fall fatality in the worst case). The Bureau of Labor Statistics (BLS) separates 'falls on the same level' from 'falls to a lower level.' In the business world workers are put at greater risk when they are required to work on a ladder or on a roof, so separating the cause of these injuries makes perfect sense. In 2011 the BLS changed the way they classify fall injuries. Falls from stairs, ladders or roofs had been identified. Starting in 2011 the BLS grouped falls to a lower level by the height of the fall instead of by the event causing the fall. The BLS also added a classification for "falls on same level while climbing stairs, steps, or curbs."

Falls vs. fall injuries

One of the problems with data is that we can only analyze the information captured. We don't know how often people actually fall. The CDC and the BLS look at the number of injuries caused by falls, but neither tracks the actual number of falls that occur either at work or in everyday life. And, quite honestly, I'm not sure how we could accurately track the number of falls that occur. The information related to how often people fall is almost anecdotal. The CDC says that one in three elderly Americans will fall each year, but the source of that information isn't documented.[24] There are many studies that look at falls in the elderly, but few on how often everyone else falls. I did find two studies that look at how the non-elderly fall, but their methodology and conclusions were very different.

The first study is from the National Institute on Aging, published in 2005, which had 1,497 participants ranging in age from 20 to 92. In this study, participants filled out a questionnaire designed to determine whether they had fallen during the last two years, and the circumstances and resulting injuries

---

24   Centers for Disease Control and Prevention, Home and Recreational Safety, http://www.cdc.gov/homeandrecreationalsafety/falls/adultfalls.html.

from those falls.[25] One of the conclusions from this study was that as we age, we fall more frequently: 18 percent of participants in the 20–45 age group reported falling during the previous two years; 21 percent in the 46–65 age group reported falling during the previous two years; and 35 percent over age 65 reported falling during the previous two years.

Then there's a 2015 study by Purdue University that tracked ninety-four underclassmen (average age of 20) by asking them to respond to a daily e-mail reporting their STF activity for the previous 24 hours.[26] In this study, which ran only sixteen weeks (30 percent of the year), researchers found that 52 percent of the participants reported that they fell at least once. That shows a much larger fall number in a much younger population—not what you might expect.

How do we reconcile these two studies? I think the difference in results is due to the methodology and how people remember a fall. For example, say it's the middle of winter and a small snowstorm has just ended. You head out to shovel your walk. On the way out, you hit a slippery patch and fall down. You're wearing a big puffy coat and you fall in a pile of fresh, soft snow. No harm done. You get up, brush yourself off, and proceed to shovel your walk. That fall is a non-event. Without a reason to make that fall memorable, it will quickly fade from your mind. If you recorded falls daily like the participants in the Purdue study, you'd be likely to remember the tumble in the driveway. Would you remember that fall when filling out a questionnaire six months or a year later? Probably not, unless there was something special about it, like an injury.

The problem is that falls are different. There's a randomness to STF injuries—with every fall, there's a risk of injury. You'll fall many times during your life. The likelihood of an injury from a fall depends on where you fall, how you fall, and how old you are. The most frequent injuries are contusions

25   Laura Talbot, et al., "Falls in Young, Middle-Aged and Older Community Dwelling Adults: Perceived Cause, Environmental Factors and Injury," *BMC Public Health* 5, no. 86 (2005), doi: 10.1186/1471-2458-5-86.

26   Michel Johannes Hubertus Heijnen and Shirley Rietdyk, "Falls in Young Adults: Perceived Causes and Environmental Factors Assessed with a Daily Online Survey," *Human Movement Science* 46 (April 2016): 86–95, doi: 10.1016/j.humov.2015.12.007.

(bruises), lacerations (cuts or gashes), broken bones, and head injuries. We know that falls are the number one cause of emergency room visits every year and for a fall to prompt an emergency room visit, it has to result in a pretty serious injury. We know that falls are the number one cause of traumatic brain injuries. We know that falls are the number one cause of accidental death for seniors. And we also know that everyone falls. What we don't know is whether your next fall will be the one that sends you to the emergency room. The best way to prevent an STF injury is to avoid a fall. Understanding why we fall can reduce the risk, so now let's examine the technical side of falls.

Slip or trip

We've already defined a fall as losing your balance and hitting the ground or another object on the way down. Falls are classified as one of two types: falls at the same level and falls from elevation or to a lower level. As we noted, most falls occur at the same level. This is because we spend most of our time walking on a level surface and we naturally become more cautious when we're dealing with steps or ladders. Not surprisingly, more serious injuries occur at elevation.

Falls happen when you lose your balance, but what does that mean? A simple way to describe losing your balance is when your center of gravity is no longer centered over your legs. Most of the time falls are caused by a slip or a trip. A slip is defined as when there's little or no friction between the floor and your foot. People slip on snow and ice, on wet surfaces or from spills, when there are changes in slope, when there are changes in the walking surfaces (such as rugs to tile).

Slips or the risk of a slip can be measured using the "coefficient of friction" between the walking surface and your foot or footwear. The higher the amount of resistance (or greater the coefficient of friction) that occurs between your foot or footwear and the walking surface, the less likely you are to slip. There are machines (tribometers) and methodologies that will accurately measure the amount of friction between the walking surface and the type, material, and design of your footwear.[27] If you're obsessive-compulsive in this area of your life, or if you're responsible for preventing falls by others at your workplace, this measurement methodology can help determine if you have a walking surface that is generally safe in many different circumstances. Things like the weather, changes in temperature, spills that aren't cleaned up, leaks from mechanical sources (anything from a refrigeration unit to a vehicle), type of footwear worn, and unsecured rugs or mats all contribute to the risk of a fall due to slipping.

On a side note, did you know that you're less likely to slip in extremely cold conditions than in temperatures closer to freezing? In my youth, when I started playing hockey, my dad taught me that ice skating wasn't possible on ice alone. The blades on my ice skates would only slip when they created enough friction to turn the ice under the blades into water. That layer of water on the ice allows the ice skates to slide smoothly over the ice. The same is true when you slip on snow or ice; it's that thin layer of water that causes the problem. Be extra careful when temperatures are just close to freezing because that's when slip hazards on ice are most likely to occur.

A trip occurs when your foot catches on or strikes an object, causing you to lose your balance. Trips happen when your momentum is moving you (and your center of gravity) forward, but an obstruction prevents your legs from staying under your center of gravity, causing you to fall. People trip on clutter, uneven walkways or sidewalks, unseen objects and obstacles, cords and cables, open file cabinet drawers, damaged carpet or walk surfaces, unmarked changes in elevation, objects protruding from a walking surface, curb drops, and wrinkled, curled, or improperly laid floor mats. A trip hazard is defined as a vertical change in elevation over one-quarter of an inch. That's not very much—about the width of a pencil.

We all live our lives with certain expectations. When these expectations aren't met, accidents occur. Traffic moves on green lights and stops at red lights. Try not stopping for a red light. The same rules apply to trips. We don't watch each and every step we take. We assume that the path we've taken in the

---

27 For an in-depth discussion of tribometers, see chapter 4 of *Slip, Trip, and Fall Prevention: A Practical Handbook* by Steven Di Pilla (Boca Raton, Florida: CRC Press, 2010).

past will be the same each time we walk it. Trips often occur when our path does not meet that expectation. Some of the leading causes of trip hazards include clutter left in a normally clear walkway or when someone leaves a lower file drawer open at shin level; unexpected changes in elevation including unmarked broken or damaged pavement; extension cords or cables placed across a walkway. The risk of tripping can be increase when there are visual obstructions like when we carry a large package or in poor lighting situations.

We can trip at any age, however, we're more likely to trip as we get older. This is due to the changes in our gait (our walk and step pattern) and muscle structure. As we get older, we tend to not lift our feet as much as we did when we were younger. If you watch, you'll notice that as people age they shuffle instead of stepping. This shuffling means they're more likely to catch their toes on smaller changes in elevations.

Now the question that must be on your mind is whether more injuries are caused by slips or trips. The BLS has captured this data for us. Figure 3.2 shows that slips cause slightly more injuries, both when there's no fall (53 percent) and when there's a fall on the same level (58 percent).

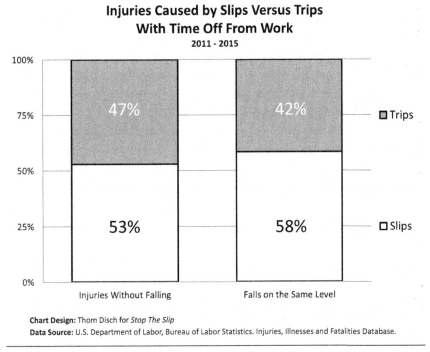

FIGURE 3.2 Injuries caused by slips vs. trips with time off from work, 2011-2015

Time for a pop quiz: Your son leaves his small toy truck in the hallway. You come out of the bathroom and step on it and fall down. Was this a slip or a trip? The answer is that it doesn't matter. The problem is that you fell. The toy truck should not have been in the hallway. In the real world, it doesn't matter whether it was slip or trip. We all need to make fall prevention a priority.

Elementary School

I was leaving my daughter's elementary school. My mind was on the conversation I'd just had with the principal and one of her teachers. It was actually a good report: my daughter, who is typically pretty shy, was starting to come out of her shell and become more active in class. I was quite proud of her. I walked out the door on my way to the parking lot and literally fell out of the building.

My daughter's elementary school was built in the 1960s, and has been modified to keep up with the times. The entryway is locked and has a camera and an intercom that requires you to identify yourself before you can enter. The odd thing about this entryway is that as soon as you open the door you have to take a step up to enter the building. This isn't a problem as you enter the building. You can clearly see the step when you open the door and you have to be buzzed in before you can enter. The combined actions of waiting for the buzzer and opening the door help you to pay attention to the step up.

It's unclear if this entryway was part of the original design or if it had been modified as a part a building modernization program. Either way, the current entryway design is a departure from standard building design. A standard design has a level walkway on both sides of a door. This is our expectation because it's the way almost all buildings are constructed. This unexpected departure from standard design was the cause of my problem.

When leaving the school there was no need to pause and talk with the office staff, so I just continued out and on my way. The problem was that I needed to remember that there was a step down once I walked out the door. I didn't remember. The principal and the superintendent both saw my fall and came to my rescue. Other than feeling clumsy and being embarrassed, I was fine.

This led to a discussion and it turned out that I wasn't the only person surprised by this step down. In fact, the superintendent herself had actually fallen out the door and injured herself earlier in the year. What I found to be the most interesting part of this story was that even though this problem was recurring and the people closest to the problem knew it was a problem, no action had been taken to eliminate the problem. There are two reasons why this problem wasn't addressed and they both go to why slips, trips, and falls are such a chronic problem. First, people saw this as an STF problem, but they saw it as a problem only for themselves. They blamed their own clumsiness and didn't want to highlight their own perceived clumsiness in front of others. Second, no one saw a quick and easy way to solve the problem. The perfect solution would have been to rebuild the entrance, but that would have been very expensive and the funds weren't in the budget.

My accident brought the problem into an open forum. Everyone agreed that this was an STF hazard and that it was a problem that needed to be addressed. We quickly realized that to solve the problem we simply needed to eliminate the step up/step down at the entryway door. So my company built a small platform outside the door. This eliminated the surprise step down problem and virtually eliminated the STF hazard. The cost of fixing it was under $2,000 and it was paid out of the general building maintenance account. Sometimes elevating an STF problem to a group for discussion creates new and unique ways to solve it.

CHAPTER 4

AGE AND FALLS

We all fall. In fact, I'm quite certain we fall a lot more than we're willing to admit. Remember this comment from the CDC: "One out of three older people falls each year."[28] It is perhaps the most frequently cited comment on falls. When I first heard it I thought, that's a lot of falls, but I had no way to put this number into perspective. Is it actually a lot?

My perspective changed when I came across the 2015 study of undergraduate students (around 20 years old) at Purdue University that had them report daily on their STF activity. This study found that over half of the participants fell at least once during the sixteen weeks of the study.[29] Yikes! This means that that youth fall a lot more than the elderly. Shirley Rietdyk, a professor of health and kinesiology who conducted the study, explained it this way, "The fall rate may be lower for older adults because they're more cautious due to the higher risk of serious, even fatal, injuries from falls."[30]

---

28   Centers for Disease Control and Prevention, Home and Recreational Safety,
      http://www.cdc.gov/homeandrecreationalsafety/falls/adultfalls.html.

29   Michel Johannes Hubertus Heijnen and Shirley Rietdyk, "Falls in Young Adults: Perceived Causes
      and Environmental Factors Assessed with a Daily Online Survey," *Human Movement Science* 46
      (April 2016): 86–95, doi: 10.1016/j.humov.2015.12.007.

30   Amy Patterson Neubert, "Don't Let Youth Trip You; More than 50 Percent Young Adults
      Fall, Trip," Purdue University News, March 9, 2016, https://www.purdue.edu/newsroom/
      releases/2016/Q1/dont-let-youth-trip-you-more-than-50-percent-young-adults-fall,-trip.html.

Let's take this to the next level: how do STF injuries relate to age? I was surprised to learn that falls create more emergency room visits for children (age 18 and younger) than for the elderly (age 65 and older). However, the bigger story is that the older we get, the more serious the consequences of a fall. When we compare the number of emergency room visits caused by falls to the number of people who die from STF injuries, falls cause approximately 2.5 million emergency room visits for both youth and the elderly (Figure 4.1). However, we find that those 2.5 million injuries cause dramatically more hospitalizations and deaths among older people.

Fall Related ER Visits, Hospitalizations and Deaths
In 2013

Age	Emergency Room Visits	Hospitalizations	Deaths
18 and Under	2,504,062	46,427	134
65 and Older	2,495,806	657,843	25,593

Data Source: NEISS All Injury Program operated by the Consumer Product Safety Commission (CPSC). National Center for Injury Prevention and Control, CDC using WISQARS™.

FIGURE 4.1 Fall-related emergency room visits, hospitalizations, and deaths, 2013

How do falls compare to other causes of emergency room visits for each age? We charted the top five reasons people visited the emergency room by age. We already knew that falls were the number one cause of emergency room visits overall, but Figure 4.2 shows that falls never ranked below number three for any age and that was only for a short period of life.

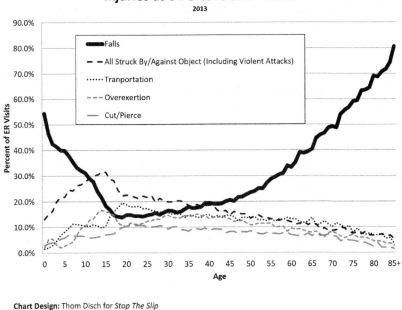

Injuries as a Percent of ER Visits
2013

Chart Design: Thom Disch for *Stop The Slip*
Data Source: NEISS All Injury Program operated by the Consumer Product Safety Commission (CPSC). National Center for Injury Prevention and Control, CDC using WISQARS™.

FIGURE 4.2 Injuries as a percentage of emergency room visits, 2013

The conclusion is that *everyone* is at risk for STF injuries. We all need to guard against falls, but we need to be especially vigilant in guarding against falls with the elderly because if they're injured in a fall, they'll be more seriously injured.

What does this pattern of STF injuries mean for us as we go through life? We charted the number of injuries per one thousand people for each age. Figure 4.3 shows that the young and the old are most at risk for STF injuries. We then applied a narrative to the reasons for this distribution of STF injuries.

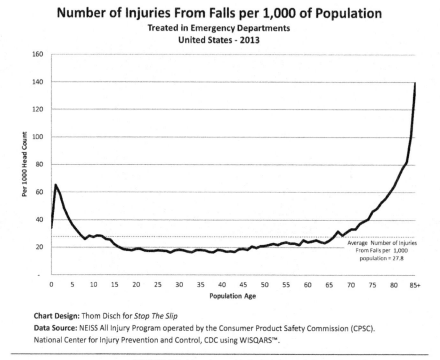

Number of Injuries From Falls per 1,000 of Population
Treated in Emergency Departments
United States - 2013

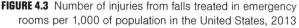

Average Number of Injuries
From Falls per 1,000
population = 27.8

Chart Design: Thom Disch for *Stop The Slip*
Data Source: NEISS All Injury Program operated by the Consumer Product Safety Commission (CPSC).
National Center for Injury Prevention and Control, CDC using WISQARS™.

FIGURE 4.3 Number of injuries from falls treated in emergency
rooms per 1,000 of population in the United States, 2013

From birth until our mid-teens, we're at a higher risk of STF injury, then that risk increases again as we approach our late sixties. The explanation for this is that we start out in life being carried by our parents. Carrying children increases the likelihood that parents will slip, trip, and fall, and when child and parent fall, children are more likely to be hurt. As children become independent and learn to walk, they will fall down more frequently and learn to gain their balance. Some of these falls will require emergency room attention, as children may fall down stairs or incur other serious injuries. As they grow older, they gain their balance but engage in other risky behaviors as they learn their physical limitations. As they hit their mid-teens, their coordination, balance, and judgment all improve. Fall injuries decrease, but they never drop below sixteen emergency room visits per year per one thousand people.

As we get into our late forties, fall injuries begin to increase. This is a natural result of the aging process. We become less physically fit. We add a few extra pounds, our coordination declines, and our vision starts to fail. Other medical conditions affect our balance and we start to take more medications that can affect our stability. At the same time, as we age, our ability to avoid a fall declines and the consequences of falls create more serious injuries; this may increase the need to go to the emergency room after a fall.

Here's a surprising fact: in 2013, if you were unfortunate enough to have died at age 21, you were just as likely to have died from a fall as someone who died at age 79.[31]

I'm guessing that your first reaction is skepticism, so let me put it a different way:

- 1.3 percent of all the people who died at age 21 died as a consequence of a fall injury.
- 1.3 percent of all the people who died at age 79 died as a consequence of a fall injury.

Shocked? I certainly was. In fact, in 2013, falls caused 1.2 percent of all deaths in the United States. Figure 4.4 shows the percentage of deaths caused by falls at each age that year.

---

31   Centers for Disease Control and Prevention, National Center for Injury Prevention and Control, Consumer Product Safety Commission, National Electronic Injury Surveillance System—All Injury Program, http://www.cdc.gov/ncipc/wisqars/nonfatal/datasources.htm. Analysis and calculations prepared by Thom Disch.

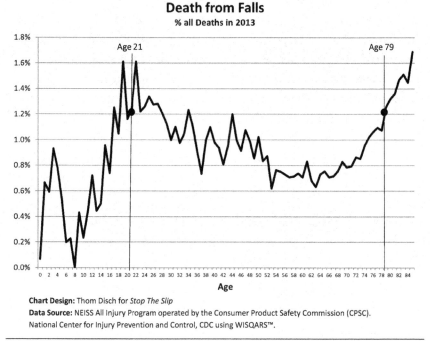

Death from Falls
% all Deaths in 2013

Chart Design: Thom Disch for *Stop The Slip*
Data Source: NEISS All Injury Program operated by the Consumer Product Safety Commission (CPSC).
National Center for Injury Prevention and Control, CDC using WISQARS™.

FIGURE 4.4 Percentage of deaths from falls by age, 2013

Once we reach adulthood, the percentage doesn't change very much. Everything we've been taught about slips, trips, and falls tell us that seniors are at a greater risk for STF injuries and deaths. So how do we explain this surprisingly high death toll from falls for everyone?

Figure 4.5 will help you understand.

Comparison of Deaths from Falls in 2013

	Age 21	Age 79
Total Population at this age	4,569,000	1,321,000
Total who died at this age	3,683	58,597
Total who died from falls	46	736
Fall deaths as a percent of total deaths	1.25%	1.26%

Calculations and Analysis: Thom Disch for *Stop The Slip*
Data Source: NEISS All Injury Program operated by the Consumer Product Safety Commission (CPSC). National Center for Injury Prevention and Control, CDC using WISQARS™.

FIGURE 4.5 Comparison of deaths from falls by age, 2013

Not very many people die at age 21. People at age 79 are much more likely to die than those at age 21. That's consistent with the cycle of life. And more people at age 79 die as a consequence of a fall—no surprise there. What is surprising is that while death is less likely at age 21, falls cause more than 1 percent of all those deaths. These mortality numbers reinforce our concern that falls are very dangerous for all adult age groups.

Consider the following statistics about children and STF injuries:

- Falls cause more than half of all nonfatal injuries to children under one year of age.[32]
- While small children can be resilient in recovering from a fall, an infant can suffer a deadly impact to the head from a fall of just 30 inches. That's about the distance from the top of a mattress to the floor.
- For children up to age 15, falls were the leading cause of emergency room visits (nonfatal injuries).[33]

---

32   Centers for Disease Control and Prevention, *CDC Childhood Injury Report* (2008), http://www.cdc.gov/safechild/Child_Injury_Data.html.
33   Ibid.

- For teenagers between 15 and 19, falls were one of the top three leading causes of nonfatal injuries.[34]
- In a typical year, over ninety thousand children under age 5 are treated at an emergency room for falling down the stairs.[35] This represents an amazing 88 percent of emergency room visits.
- Other than children falling down the stairs on their own, carrying children down the stairs is the next most common cause of children on stairs injuries, resulting in five thousand child injuries a year.[36]

Erin and Josh

Erin is the youngest of three siblings and the last to start a family. Her pregnancy and delivery were textbook—not a single day with morning sickness, and no complications. Her sister and sister-in-law both claimed to be terribly jealous. Now baby Josh was three months old and she was taking him on his first real field trip: Erin's brother had just bought a new house and the whole family was gathering there to see the new setup.

It happened as Erin and Josh were coming down the large, curving staircase. The stairs were carpeted and the footing was good. Wanting to protect Josh, Erin held him close with both hands and started down the stairs. What actually caused the fall is unclear, but halfway down, Erin lost her footing and tumbled down the steps. The result of the emergency room visit was a cast on Josh's broken arm and lots of bruises and sore muscles for Erin.

This fall had four contributing factors:

Erin and Josh were in an unfamiliar environment.

Erin was holding Josh up high, near her face, obscuring her view of the stairs.

Because Erin was carrying Josh, her center of gravity was higher than normal, making her more unstable. The higher a person's center of gravity,

34   Ibid.

35   Ashley E. Zielinski, et al., "Stair-Related Injuries to Young Children Treated in US Emergency Departments, 1999–2008," *Pediatrics* 129, no. 4 (2012), doi: 10.1542/peds.2011-2314.

36   Ibid.

the more likely she is to fall; conversely, the lower her center of gravity, the more stable she is.

When Erin started walking down the stairs, she was using both hands to cradle Josh. This meant that she had no free hand to hold the handrail. With each step she took, she had only one point of contact for stability. When we change elevations, this single point of contact becomes more of a challenge. Use of a handrail provides two constant points of contact and increases stability.

Fall prevention for children

What could Erin have done to reduce the STF risk for herself and her son? Not taking Josh up the stairs is one option. Unfamiliar environments, combined with new or unusual conditions, such as being unused to carrying a baby around, force the mind and body to compensate for a lot of factors. Keep it simple and you'll reduce your risk.

Another thing to consider is using a baby carrier. As a parent, your first instinct is to cradle and protect your child. A carrier—there are several different versions on the market—will allow you to feel protective and still keep your hands free to hold the handrail.

Also make sure that your child isn't in a position to obstruct your view of the stairs. Because we've all walked up and down thousands of stairs, we automatically assume we know where the next step will be. In a new environment this expectation and the stairs could be off by just enough to cause an accident. Looking directly at your foot placement on the stairs will make you safer.

Of course, we want to protect our kids from injury. We teach them some basic safety precautions, like looking both ways when they cross the street and not running with sharp objects. I even remember my mom telling me not to play on the stairs. If you don't already, make it a habit to remind your children about ways to avoid an STF injury.

Here are some higher-risk situations and some actions you can take to reduce the risk of STF injuries for children:

- **Stairs:** Use approved safety gates at the tops and bottoms of stairs. Select the proper gate for your specific need and install it properly. Some gates are designed specifically to be used at the top of stairs; others are intended to be used only at the bottom of the stairs. Seek professional assistance if you have questions or need help when selecting and installing safety gates. Actively supervise toddlers on stairs. Hold their hands when walking up and down the steps.
- **Windows:** Each year over 3,300 children go to the emergency room (and about eight die) as a result of falling out of a window.[37] Screens are designed to keep bugs out, not kids in—don't count on screens to guard against a fall. Install window guards to protect children from open windows or install window stops that prevent the window from opening more than four inches. Move chairs, cribs, and other furniture away from windows to reduce children's risk of falling out of a window when they are climbing.
- **Playgrounds:** Check the surfaces under playground equipment. They should be safe, soft, and consist of appropriate materials (such as recycled rubber chips, wood chips, or sand, not concrete, asphalt, or dirt). The surface materials should be an appropriate depth and well maintained. While you can't always control the surface material at the playground, you can control which playgrounds your children use.
- **Sports and athletic activities:** When playing sports, skateboarding, rollerblading, and bike riding, make sure your children wear appropriate protective gear, especially helmets.
- **Highchairs, shopping carts, swings, and portable carriers:** Make sure that your children are securely strapped into the seat properly. Place portable carriers on the floor, not on a table or elevated surface. Make sure that your children are being watched at all times when you use these devices.

---

37 National Safety Council, "Windows Are Vital to Survival, but Keep Safety in Mind," http://www.nsc.org/learn/safety-knowledge/Pages/about-national-window-safety-week.aspx

Fall prevention for the elderly

In my research, I was surprised to find that fall injuries (as measured by emergency room visits) are spread out pretty evenly across the age groups (as can be seen in Figures 4.6 and 4.7): one quarter in children under 16, one quarter in ages 16 to 44, one quarter in ages 45 to 68, and one quarter over age 68. So why is so much written about the problem of falls and the elderly?

Fall Related ER Visits, Hospitalizations and Deaths
In 2013

Number of Incidents

Age Group	Emergency Room Visits	Hospitalizations	Deaths
Under 16	2,263,344	41,124	76
16 to 44	2,182,868	85,791	1,556
45 to 68	2,187,225	257,096	5,257
Over 68	2,156,483	597,377	24,349

Percent of Total

Age Group	Emergency Room Visits	Hospitalizations	Deaths
Under 16	25%	4%	0%
16 to 44	25%	9%	5%
45 to 68	25%	26%	17%
Over 68	25%	61%	78%

Data Source: NEISS All Injury Program operated by the Consumer Product Safety Commission (CPSC). National Center for Injury Prevention and Control, CDC using WISQARS™.

FIGURE 4.6 Table of fall injuries, hospitalizations, and deaths by age group, 2013

It turns out that fall injuries have a much greater impact on us as we get older. We're able to rebound from an STF injury when we're younger, but as we age, our ability to recover declines. Splitting the population by the age groups listed above, so that each group has approximately the same number of fall injuries, we can look at the consequences of falls as measured by hospitalizations and the resulting number of deaths for each age group. Hospitalizations and mortality from falls are quite low for the youngest age groups. While children under age 16 represent 25 percent of the emergency room visits, they represent only 4 percent of hospitalizations caused by falls, and falls caused only seventy-six deaths in this group, which is actually less than one half of 1 percent of all deaths from falls. By contrast, the over 68 group, which also had 25 percent of the emergency room visits caused by falls, had 61 percent of the hospitalizations and 78 percent of the deaths caused by falls. Figures 4.6 and 4.7 show the big picture.

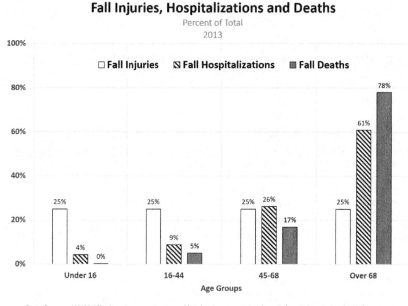

Data Source: NEISS All Injury Program operated by the Consumer Product Safety Commission (CPSC). National Center for Injury Prevention and Control, CDC using WISQARS™.

FIGURE 4.7 Chart of fall injuries, hospitalizations, and deaths by age group, 2013

As we age, we lose muscle mass and our reflexes slow down; our gait changes and we lift our feet less; our depth perception changes and our eyesight worsens; we add medications to treat new medical conditions, and that medication can affect our balance. This means that aging affects us negatively in two ways: we're less able to avoid a fall and our bodies become more fragile, resulting in more fall-related injuries. Most of the injuries caused by falls involve either broken bones or head injuries.[38] In fact, over 95 percent of all hip fractures are caused by falls.[39] Falls cause 51 percent of all traumatic brain injuries in the elderly.[40]

These changes happen gradually and we adjust our activities and our lifestyles as a result. It's all part of growing older.

There are three things you can do to reduce your risk of injury from slips, trip, and falls as you age:

- Become aware of the causes of falls, especially those that affect older adults and attend to each one as they're introduced into your life. Reading this book is a great way to see all of the fall risk factors that will affect you. Address each factor and decide how you'll minimize that risk and stay safe.

- Develop and maintain an exercise program to strengthen your leg muscles and your core and improve your balance. Two fitness programs that can help are tai chi and yoga; you can find instructors and classes online.

- Discuss your concerns with your doctor and pharmacist. They can review your medications and alert you to any possible side effects and interactions. Discussing STF risks with other family members so they can help you avoid STF risks.

One of the biggest challenges of working with the elderly is convincing them that they're at greater risk for an STF injury. We all have our blind spots. We notice other people's poor driving habits even though we make the same mistakes. When someone points out one of our mistakes, we're quick to defend

---

38 Centers for Disease Control and Prevention, National Center for Health Statistics, Health Data Interactive, www.cdc.gov/nchs/hdi.htm.

39 Wilson Hayes, et al., "Impact Near the Hip Dominates Fracture Risk in Elderly Nursing Home Residents Who Fall," *Calcified Tissue International* 52, no. 3 (1993): 192–198, doi: 10.1007/BF00298717.

40 Hilaire Thompson, et al., "Traumatic Brain Injury in Older Adults: Epidemiology, Outcomes, and Future Implications," *Journal of the American Geriatrics Society* 54, no. 10 (2006): 1590–1595, doi: 10.1111/j.1532-5415.2006.00894.x.

our actions, not because we want to deny what we did but rather because we truly believe that we were doing the right thing. This is human nature.

People who are just entering old age are often still in denial about being elderly. As a result, they may be unwilling to listen to advice relating to what older people should do. Even if they've accepted the fact that they're in the elderly category, they've been at risk for STF injuries for some time. This means that while they may welcome the advice, they may also have had an STF injury that could have been prevented if they'd had this advice earlier.

The solution is to change our approach. We know that STF injuries happen to everyone. As we've seen, 25 percent happen to people under age 16 and 25 percent happen to people over 68. The STF problem is universal. We need to begin teaching everyone about STF injuries earlier in life. Next, when approaching the elderly, our focus needs to be on how STF injuries happen to everyone and that the elderly need to be aware of fall injuries to help prevent them and protect not only themselves, but also the people they care about. This eliminates the "you're old and you need to be more careful" confrontation.

It's a simple process to modify any of the existing programs to help reduce slips, trips, and falls among the elderly. The National Council on Aging and the CDC are just two of many organizations that have developed programs to reduce falls for older adults. You can find them at these websites:

- ncoa.org/healthy-aging/falls-prevention/
- cdc.gov/homeandrecreationalsafety/falls/adultfalls.html

CHAPTER 5

FOOTWEAR

No one will make the argument that stilettos are safer than flats. And no one will tell you they're more comfortable. Yet high heels are chosen over flats every day because fashion requires it. According to a survey of three thousand women cited in *Glamour* magazine, "The average woman will buy 469 pairs of shoes in her lifetime with an overall price tag of about $25,000."[41] Each of these women has about nineteen pairs of shoes, including three pairs of heels; six pairs of flip-flops, sandals, ballet flats, and wedges; three pairs of boots; and four pairs of "foxy" shoes for nights out.

This is an entertaining side note, but what does it have to do with slips, trips, and falls? In American society, shoes are a fashion statement. And while some women elevate this to an art form, many men do the same thing. The problem is the conflict of safety versus style and fashion. Unfortunately, safety rarely wins that battle.

As we discussed earlier, slips happen when there isn't enough friction between your foot and the walking surface. A typical slip has three components: the walking surface, your footwear, and the material you slipped on. Footwear is the component that you have the most control over.

---

41   Tracey Lomrantz Lester, "The Average Woman Spends Almost $25,000 on Shoes in Her Lifetime! How About You?" *Glamour*, June 28, 2010, http://www.glamour.com/story/the-average-woman-spends-almos.

The National Floor Safety Institute published statistics on the causes of STF injuries in the food service industry (Figure 5.1).[42] This included injuries among both employees and customers. Their analysis showed that footwear caused 24 percent of STF injuries. And floor surface and footwear together caused almost three-quarters of all the STF injuries. The causes may be different outside of the food service industry, but I'm pretty sure that these two causes represent the majority of STF injuries in all aspects of our lives.

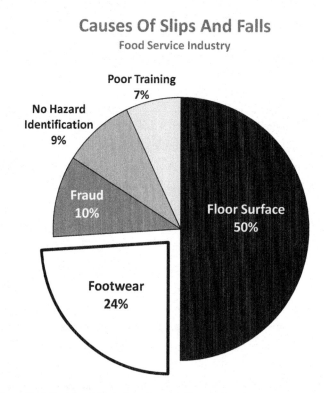

Causes Of Slips And Falls
Food Service Industry

Data Source: The National Floor Safety Institute. Restaurant Slip-and-Fall Accident Prevention Program. Produced as a part of the NFSI Best Practices Project 2003

FIGURE 5.1 Causes of slips and falls in the food service industry

42   National Floor Safety Institute, *Restaurant Slip-and-Fall Accident Prevention Program*, 2003,

Let's look at how footwear selection may increase the risk of an STF accident.

Flip-flops and sandals

Flip-flops are considered the most dangerous shoes on the market.[43] In addition to the exposure to bacteria and the lack of support, they pose an STF hazard because they change the way you walk and they rarely have a secure gripping surface. The design of flip-flops and some sandals requires you to curl your toes to keep them on your feet. This curling action changes your gait and that, in turn, increases the risk for an STF injury. [44] Even with this curling action, many people trip and fall when the flip-flop or sandal slides off their foot. Joel Greenberg, an expert on personal injury issues, says that most attorneys feel it's almost impossible to win a slip, trip, and fall lawsuit if the injured person was wearing flip-flops.[45] (We'll discuss the legal side of slips, trips, and falls in more depth in Chapter 23, "Lawsuits and Litigation.")

The UK National Health Service studied this and determined that two hundred thousand people in the United Kingdom are injured by wearing flip-flops each year, with some of the most common injuries being sprains. The agency estimates that Brits spend about £40 million per year on health care for injuries caused by wearing flip-flops.[46] One of the notable issues with flip-flops is that, unlike regular shoes with laces, flip flops aren't "locked" to the wearer's feet. As a result, when wearers turn or shift their weight, they often slip out of the shoes. The American Medical News recognized this phenomenon as a

43   Russell J. Kendzior, *Falls Aren't Funny: America's Multi-Billion Dollar Slip-and-Fall Crisis* (Rowman & Littlefield, 2010), 119.

44   Nassau Board of Cooperative Education Services, Office of the Safety Coordinator, *Footwear Safety Guidelines*, http://www.nassauboces.org/cms/lib5/ny18000988/centricity/ domain/208/safety/footwear_safety_guidelines.pdf.

45   Interview with Joel Greenburg, Chicago, July 2015. Joel H. Greenburg, Ltd.

46   Sophie Borland, "Flip-flops 'injure 200,000 a year' costing the NHS an astonishing £40m," *Daily Mail*, July 29, 2010, http://www.dailymail.co.uk/health/article-1298471/Flip-flops-injure-200-000-year-costing-NHS-astonishing-40m.html.

disturbingly common cause of metatarsal fractures[47] (also known as broken bones in the foot).

The US Consumer Product Safety Commission (CPSC) is well aware of the hazard created by flip-flops and sandals, especially when they're made a certain way. It's not uncommon to see a particular style of flip-flops or sandals recalled by the agency due to increased fall risk. For example, JP Boden recalled a pair of children's sandals in 2013 because the cork sole had a tendency to detach from the sandal, increasing the STF risk.[48] Madewell recalled a pair of women's sandals in 2015 for a similar problem. As the CPSC describes the issue, "The metal shank can dislodge and break through the bottom of the outsole, posing a fall hazard."[49] These are two among many examples that can be found on the CPSC's website. To mitigate your risk of tripping and falling because of the shoes you're wearing, clearly it's necessary to examine how a particular pair of shoes is made before you purchase them.

---

47 American Medical Association, "Flip-Flops Causing Slips and Trips—and Serious Injuries," *American Medical News*, September 3, 2007, http://www.amednews.com/article/20070903/health/309039969/6/.

48 US Consumer Product Safety Commission, "JP Boden Recalls Children's Sandals Due to Fall Hazard (Recall Alert)," August 15, 2013, https://www.cpsc.gov/Recalls/2013/jp-boden-recalls-childrens-sandals.

49 US Consumer Product Safety Commission, "Madewell Recalls Women's Sandals Due to Fall Hazard," August 20, 2015, https://www.cpsc.gov/Recalls/2015/Madewell-Recalls-Womens-Sandals/.

Brad Pitt

Actor Brad Pitt learned the hard way that flip-flops pose a serious STF hazard. In April 2015, he showed up at the third annual Light Up the Blues Concert in Hollywood with bruises all over his face. As he told *People* magazine, "This is what happens when you try to run up steps in the dark, with your hands full, wearing flip-flops. Turns out, if you then try to stop your forward momentum with your face, the result is road rash."[50] Of course, running up the stairs in the dark poses its own set of problems, even for those wearing better shoes. We'll examine that more fully in Chapter 13, "Poor Lighting and Reduced Vision."

Flip-flops can cause other problems too because they expose the feet to outside elements that can include everything from sharp objects to rain. The elements can cause the entire bottoms of your feet to start slipping as you walk. Flip-flops also lack support for the foot and arches, causing the foot to lift up as you walk. This can result in the back of the flip-flop getting stuck in things like escalators or revolving doors, leading to more serious injuries than a stubbed toe.

I realize that summer almost requires the wearing of flip-flops and sandals and I certainly don't want to anger the fashion police, so while this type of footwear is basically unsafe, consider wearing sandals with a back strap to make them safer.

Barefoot and stocking feet

The problem of improper footwear isn't isolated to the realm of flip-flops. Many of us walk around our homes either barefoot or wearing only socks. Truth be told, I'm writing this chapter in my bare feet. This, it turns out, can also increase the risk of a fall or STF injury. One study looked at the footwear

50 Amanda Michelle Steiner, "The Truth Behind Brad Pitt's Bruised Face Involves Walking in Flip Flops," *People*, April 26, 2015, http://people.com/celebrity/brad-pitt-has-a-bruised-face-at-autism-speaks-event-in-hollywood/.

of people over 65 and how this contributed to falls. This study compared three categories: wearing athletic/canvas shoes, all other shoes, and barefoot or stocking feet. After adjusting for other factors, the conclusion was that athletic/canvas shoes were the safest. Wearing other types of shoes increased your fall risk by 30 percent. Wearing no shoes at all increased your risk of a fall 11.2 times, or 1,120 percent.[51] I think I'm going to put on a pair of shoes.

In all seriousness, you're eight to eleven times more likely to fall when you're *not* wearing shoes than when you are wearing shoes. There are three contributing factors to this conclusion: First, we do some of our riskier behavior without shoes, like showering. Second, without shoes, the feet are more vulnerable to painful trauma if an unexpected obstacle is encountered and this can result in a fall. And third, stocking feet may provide a poor coefficient of friction and thus be more prone to slipping. Just think about the last time you went down hardwood stairs in only your stocking feet.

Leather soles

If you've ever shopped for high-quality leather shoes, you've probably noticed that most high-end shoes have leather soles. If you've ever owned leather-soled shoes you know that they're an STF hazard. Leather soles are very slippery—on both hard surfaces and on carpet—because they're polished and have no tread pattern to minimize STF risks. Furthermore, they're noisier to walk in and they wear out more quickly. So why are leather soles so popular? I went on a quest to find out the benefits of leather soles.

It seems that the number one reason for having leather soles is tradition. This is true for both women and men. The fashionistas say things like leather soles breathe better and form more closely to your foot, and how stupid it is to even think about wearing rubber soles or rubber overlays on your soles. One pundit even said that wearing rubber-soled shoes was like wearing a dress shirt with a pocket. (As a side note, without a pocket, I have no idea where I would put my pocket protector.)

---

51   Thomas Koepsell, et al., "Footwear Style and Risk of Falls in Older Adults," *Journal of the American Geriatrics Society* 52, no. 9 (2004), 1495–1501, doi: 10.1111/j.1532-5415.2004.52412.x.

By now it's clear that I'm not the most fashion-conscious person out there. But from a practical perspective, there are a lot of shoes that have discreet, non-slip rubber overlays that provide a tremendous improvement in safety. For most of us, the well-designed rubber overlay isn't noticeable. Some shoemakers, while not embracing the full non-slip concept, have incorporated a rubber non-slip heel onto a shoe that otherwise has a leather sole. While not perfect, this does improve safety.

High heels

Anyone who has worn high heels knows the risk of tripping and falling. It's not uncommon for the heels to break off, causing the wearer to stumble. Heels can get caught on something, like a bump in the sidewalk. They can get stuck in a soft surface like wet grass, which can pull the shoe off, causing a tumble. In 2012, Australian Prime Minister Julia Gillard told the media that she fell after her heel got stuck in wet grass, pulling her shoe off. When she took her next step without her shoe, she ended up falling.

High heels naturally throw the wearer off balance, as evidenced by the wobbly gait of first-time wearers. Heels put much more pressure on the ankles than most wearers are used to dealing with, which is why people trying to walk in high heels for the first time are so unsteady. Their ankles are unable to meet the demand the shoes place on their joints. But even women who wear high heels daily are at risk of stumbling and falling, as demonstrated by the many videos, photos, and articles reporting on models or celebrities falling while wearing high heels.

It's possible to fracture your foot due to a fall while wearing high heels, according to Dr. Neal M. Blitz. In a *Huffington Post* article, he explained, "The higher the heel and skinnier the stiletto, the more likely one is for a fall—especially on uneven terrain."[52]

The best way to avoid falling in high heels is to not wear them. Okay, now that you've stopped laughing, I'll admit that I can't give serious advice to high

---

[52] Neal M. Blitz, "The High Heel Foot Fracture: A Real Injury," *Huffington Post,* August 25, 2012, http://www.huffingtonpost.com/neal-m-blitz/high-heel-foot-injury_b_1622464.html

heel wears because I have no idea what it's like to wear them. Professional models fall when wearing high heels, so you know it will happen. I know there are hundreds of videos on YouTube that will tell you how to walk in heels and many of them have conflicting methods for avoiding a fall. You have to learn what's right for you. Limit the height of the shoe heel and the size of the heel to something you're comfortable with. And, like everything else, practice makes perfect.

Tips for choosing safe shoes

We've now looked at several versions of what *not* to wear, but what *should* you wear to prevent slips, trips, and falls? You'll need to select the best shoe for the situation. Remember that most falls connected to footwear are caused by slips, and that slips occur when there's not enough friction between your foot or footwear and the walking surface. But what kind of shoes to choose?

The three characteristics of a safe shoe are:

- A slip-resistant sole includes some form of rubberized material and a non-slip pattern. There are many different types of non-slip patterns. The key to a good non-slip pattern is adequate channeling that lets liquid flow out from the sole, allowing the sole to make solid contact with the walking surface and preventing hydroplaning. Figure 5.2 shows some non-slip patterns for different types of shoes.

Shoe Print for Non-Slip Patterns

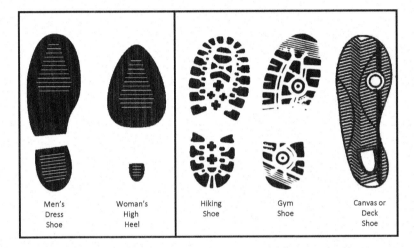

FIGURE 5.2 Shoe prints for nonslip patterns

- The safest shoe has a low heel and a solid, wide base for stability.
- A safe shoe has a strong heel pocket and laces up securely, keeping the foot securely in the shoe and protecting it from rolling over in uneven terrain.

If you're choosing shoes for work, you'll want to add other safety features that are specific to your job, such as steel toes, but that isn't tied to STF injuries.

CHAPTER 6

WEATHER

Does winter increase the number of injuries and deaths caused by falling? My first reaction to this question was, of course it does, but then I dug into the numbers. I found that the data doesn't support that contention. That's not to say that ice and snow *don't* cause fall injuries—they do. But there are so many other causes of STF injuries and deaths that ice and snow don't appear to be a primary cause. You're probably skeptical, so let me show you how I came to this remarkable conclusion.

In its 2015 *Injury Facts* report, the National Safety Council (NSC) reported the number of deaths per month for specific types of accidents in 2011 (Figure 6.1).[53] If we look at the number of deaths per day, it turns out that October was the worst month for STF deaths, even though it wasn't a particularly icy and snowy month. December came in second, but the dead of winter— January, February, and March—ranked fourth, fifth, and sixth, respectively. If ice and snow were the leading causes of falls resulting in death, we would expect the winter months to be the worst for deaths from falls. Surprisingly, this wasn't true.

---

53   National Safety Council, *Injury Facts*, 2015 edition: 23, http://www.nsc.org/Membership%20 Site%20Document%20Library/2015%20Injury%20Facts/NSC_InjuryFacts2015Ed.pdf.

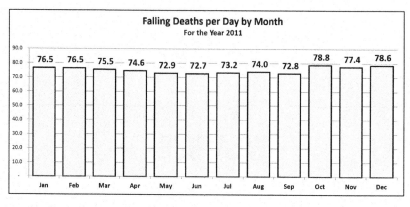

Data Source: National Safety Council, 2015 Injury Facts. Data from National Center for Health Statistics–Mortality Data for 2011, as compiled from data provided by the 57 vital statistics jurisdictions through the Vital Statistics Cooperative Program.

FIGURE 6.1 Falling deaths per day by month, 2011

That led me to question the data. The NSC and the National Center for Health Statistics are tremendously reliable. What should seasonality look like? Let's look at deaths from falls by month for two causes of death that may also have seasonal trends: drowning, which you would expect to go up in the summer months when more people are swimming, and deaths from fire or smoke, which you would expect to go up in winter, when people do unsafe things to keep warm. In Figure 6.2 there's obvious seasonality for both drowning and fire/smoke deaths, but we essentially find only slight variations in deaths by month for falls.

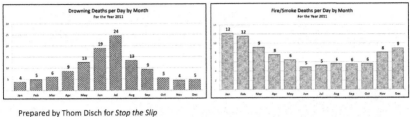

Prepared by Thom Disch for *Stop the Slip*
Data Source: National Safety Council analysis of National Center for Health Statistics–Mortality Data for 2011, as compiled from data provided by the 57 vital statistics jurisdictions through the Vital Statistics Cooperative Program.

FIGURE 6.2 Deaths per day by month – Drowning and Smoke/Fire, 2011

Similar numbers aren't available for injuries, but I think we can use deaths as a good representation of the issue.

Do you believe me yet? Let's cut the data another way. The Centers for Disease Control and Prevention have compiled data on falls as a cause of death in each US state. If the ice and snow are a dominant cause of STF injuries and deaths, those states that experience the worst ice and snow will also have the most deaths caused by falls. Let's start off comparing the states that have perhaps the worst and best weather conditions: Alaska and Hawaii. In Alaska, 4.05 people out of every one hundred thousand will die from an STF injury. In Hawaii, 8.59 people out of every one hundred thousand die from an STF injury. Yes, you read that correctly: Hawaii, with its nearly perfect weather, has more than twice as many people dying from falls as Alaska. Figure 6.3 shows US states ranked by their death rate from falls.[54]

---

54   Centers for Disease Control and Prevention, Fatal Injury Mapping, https://wisqars.cdc.gov:8443/cdcMapFramework/.

States Ranked by Number of Deaths Caused by Falls per 100K of Population
For Years: 2008-2010

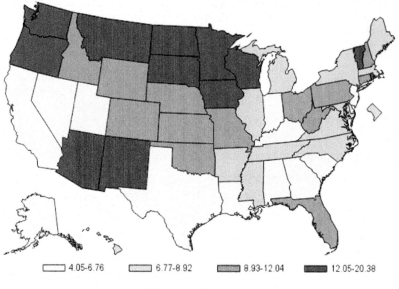

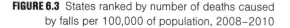

   4.05-6.76   6.77-8.92   8.93-12.04   12.05-20.38

Average Rate for US for All Three Years: 8.40

Map Produced by: The Statistics, Programming & Economics Branch, National Center of Injury Prevention & Control, CDC
Data Sources: NCES National Vital Statistics System for numbers of deaths; US Census Bureau for Population

FIGURE 6.3 States ranked by number of deaths caused by falls per 100,000 of population, 2008–2010

Some patterns can be attributed to the colder weather. In general, northern states have more STF deaths than southern states. However, in addition to the Alaska/Hawaii contrast, I find it surprising that states in the same vicinity have very different fall risks: Ohio versus Indiana, Vermont versus Maine, and New Mexico versus Utah.

So there must be some other contributing factor. Maybe age? We ran the same analysis for people under age 65. The map remained essentially the same, with very similar contradictions. We even tried to run some sophisticated modeling programs like regression analysis to determine a statistical correlation for fall injuries with age and temperature by state, but we couldn't find a strong enough relationship to draw any solid conclusions. Intuitively, we know that ice and snow cause more falls and more injuries and deaths. We also know that we're more susceptible to serious fall injuries and deaths as we age, yet we couldn't build a model to depict this. This was very confusing, but then I realized that this very confusion was the conclusion:

Falls, fall injuries, and fall deaths are complex, with multiple causes. The only way to protect ourselves and our loved ones from this risk is to increase our awareness of the variety of causes that lead to fall injuries, and deaths.

That complexity is why this is a book and not just a pamphlet telling you to avoid snow and ice and to be more careful as you get older. So how else does weather increase STF risk? Two other factors come into play: moisture and temperature.

Jim

It was a dark and stormy night when the sump pump went out. It had been a wet and rainy fall, and the sump pump had been running pretty much constantly for the past week. Through a creative usage of bath towels and rags, Jim was able to contain the seepage and avoid water damage in the basement. The next morning, he called a local plumber and had them evaluate the problem. Diagnosis? The sump pump needed to be replaced. Jim gave the okay and headed into work.

The plumber replaced the broken pump and put the old one outside, next to the garbage can by the garage, so Jim could inspect it when he arrived home that evening.

Because he got into the office late, Jim worked late that night. When he got home it was already dark. He noticed a stream of water running across the driveway, creating a puddle. Following the water trail, he saw the pump sitting next to the garage. He thought about taking a quick look before he threw it in the trash, but since the pump wasn't going anywhere and he was tired, he decided to look at the pump later in the week.

As always happens when fall turns into winter, the temperature drops below freezing and this was the first night this year that it got that cold. When Jim woke up the next morning, he completely forgot about the broken sump pump. With his mind on the workday ahead, he headed out to his car and walked across the driveway.

Jim's wife, Patti, saw it happen from the kitchen window and immediately called 911. He was just walking to the garage like any other morning, but when he hit the ice that formed where the puddle had been the previous night, his legs went out from under him and he fell backward, hitting his head on the driveway. The paramedics took him to the hospital, where he was diagnosed with a subdural hematoma or bleeding on the brain. Jim awoke from a coma four days later.

Moisture can take several forms in nature: we've already talked about ice and snow, but there's also rain, high humidity, dew, and frost. Water makes things more slippery; it acts as a lubricant between the walking surface and your foot. That's obvious. Temperature adds additional risk. When it approaches freezing, water gets more slippery. Also obvious. But what about high humidity and warm temperatures? This combination creates the perfect outdoor conditions for mold and mildew to grow on decks, stairs, walking paths, and boardwalks. If you live in an environment like this, you realize two things: one, it's very slippery and two, they grow slowly over time and can be camouflaged right on your walking path and stairway. My company has seen this in Oregon and in Washington State, where our HandiTreads™⁵⁵ have frequently been installed to combat this very problem.

Be especially careful on asphalt driveways and walkways when it begins raining. Oils naturally rise to the surface of asphalt when it's sunny and warm. This combination of water and oil is especially slippery. The risk declines after the rain has fallen for a while, the oils will wash away.

I have an electronic outdoor thermometer that flashes a warning when the temperature nears the freezing point. This is a great reminder to be cautious when going outside. Walk around any high-risk areas. And, once again, if you must walk through a high-risk area, take smaller steps, expect it to be slippery and use caution. If this is a recurring problem area, apply a non-slip treatment.

---

55   HandiTreads: are an aluminum embossed tread that can be screwed down to outside stairs and
        walkways to reduce the risk of slip and fall injuries; www.handitreads.com.

CHAPTER 7

MEDICATIONS, ALCOHOL, AND RECREATIONAL DRUGS

Everyone reacts differently to medications, alcohol, and recreational drugs. Misuse or unexpected reactions to any of these is classified by the Centers for Disease Control and Prevention (CDC) as poisoning. Over 95 percent of all poisonings in the United States are caused by the body's reaction to medications, alcohol, and recreational drugs.[56]

This classification of poisoning is the only accidental cause of death that has grown faster than falls, although there may be some ambiguity between the cause of an accident for these two categories. For example, if a person drinks too much and is injured in a fall (or worse), the accident could be classified as a consequence of either poisoning or a fall, depending on the box checked by the medical personnel who fill out the form.

---

56   Centers for Disease Control and Prevention, National Center for Injury Prevention and Control, https://webappa.cdc.gov/sasweb/ncipc/leadcaus10_us.html, Analysis of unintentional poisoning deaths by ICD codes performed by Thom Disch.

Diane

Diane is a smart, pretty twenty-four-year-old with a positive outlook and an active social life. There's just one thing that nags at her: she's convinced that her nose is too big. Even though her friends and family tell her she doesn't need a nose job, Diane is unconvinced.

Diane sees an opportunity when she visits her doctor for a sinus infection and he tells her that she has a deviated septum. After a little research, Diane finds that she can combine a rhinoplasty (or nose job) with her deviated septum surgery. She finds a great plastic surgeon and schedules a date for the operation.

Diane follows all the prep rules and arrives at the hospital. She's a bundle of nerves, but she completes the admission forms and reads all the information she's given, including a warning about the postsurgical effects of the anesthesia. But she can't really concentrate on what's being said—she just wants to get past the procedure. Thankfully, the surgery is successful, with no complications.

When Diane wakes up in her room post-surgery, she looks around but doesn't see anyone. She's a little groggy, but the most urgent thing on her mind is that she has to pee. She sees the call button for the nurse. Didn't they say something about calling the nurse when she woke up? But that's not right. She decides to call the nurse when she gets out of the bathroom. So she pulls back the covers, turns, sits up, and puts her feet on the floor. Her head spins a little bit, but it passes quickly, so she pushes off and starts making her way to bathroom.

The nurse making her rounds peeks into Diane's room and is surprised to find the bed empty. She glances down the hall but doesn't see her patient. She steps further in the room and finds Diane sprawled on the floor and bleeding. Diane forgot that she'd been warned not to get up on her own after surgery. In her effort to be self-sufficient, she passed out and fell on her new nose.

Diane is checked for other injuries, but it looks like her nose is the primary concern. The surgical team is reassembled and they go about repairing the damage caused by her fall.

We're susceptible to STF injuries when we least expect it. Medications, alcohol, and other drugs affect our balance and our ability to react to STF risks. To complicate things, there's no way to predict how you'll be affected by a change in your medications. Keep this additional risk in mind whenever you're using any chemicals that might affect your balance or reaction time. We'll split the discussion of prevention into two categories: recreation and medication.

Recreation: We all know that alcohol and recreational drugs affect our coordination and balance. You can experience a loss of personal control that may lead to an injury. The best advice is the tagline on every beer commercial: Please use responsibly.

Medication: For the purposes of this book, medications include all prescription and over-the-counter drugs, dietary supplements, vitamins, botanicals, minerals, and herbal remedies. Medications may interact with each other, as well as with alcohol, recreational drugs, food, or even your body's natural chemistry, resulting in increased STF risk. Use extreme caution when you add or change your medications, and always consult a medical professional.

The Food and Drug Administration (FDA) has developed these tips about drug interactions:[57]

- **Drug-drug interactions** happen when two or more medicines react with one another to cause unwanted effects. This kind of interaction can also cause one medicine to not work as well or even make one medicine stronger than it should be. For example, you should not take aspirin if you're on a prescription blood thinner, such as warfarin, unless directed by your health care professional.
- **Drug-condition interactions** happen when a medical condition you already have makes certain drugs potentially harmful. For example, if you have high blood pressure or asthma, you could have an unwanted reaction if you take a nasal decongestant.
- **Drug-food interactions** result from drugs reacting with foods or drinks. In some cases, food in the digestive tract can affect how a drug is absorbed. Some medicines also may affect the way nutrients are absorbed or used in the body.
- **Drug-alcohol interactions** can happen when the medicine you take reacts with an alcoholic drink. For instance, mixing alcohol with some medicines may cause you to feel tired and slow your reactions.

As we age, many of us take more medications. This, combined with the changes that our bodies go through as part of aging, can result in drug interactions that increase STF risk. Also keep in mind that some problems you might think are medicine-related, such as loss of coordination, memory loss, or irritability, could be the result of a drug interaction.

Your doctor and pharmacist can help you understand the way that over-the-counter drugs and supplements may affect you. The FDA has compiled a list of questions you can use with your doctor or pharmacist when you change your medications to help you start the conversation:[58]

---

57   US Food and Drug Administration, "Drug Interactions: What You Should Know," http://www.fda.gov/drugs/resourcesforyou/ucm163354.htm.

58   Ibid.

- Can I take it with other drugs?
- Should I avoid certain foods, beverages, or other products?
- What are possible drug interaction signs I should know about?
- How will the drug work in my body?
- Is there more information available about the drug or my condition (on the Internet or in health and medical literature)?

Learn how to take drugs safely and responsibly. Remember, the drug label and inserts will tell you:

- What the drug is used for
- How to take the drug
- How to reduce the risk of drug interactions and unwanted side effects
- The possible side effects of each medication
- Possible interactions that each new medicine may have with medicines you're already taking

Figure 7.1 lists medications that increase the risk of slips, trips, and falls.[59]

---

59   University of Nebraska Medical Center, "Table of Medications that Increase Fall Risk," 2013, http://www.unmc.edu/patient-safety/_documents/meds-with-fall-risk-brand-generic-table-2013.pdf.

Table of Medications that Increase Fall Risk

Drug Type	Drug Class	Risk Factor
Antidiabetic agents	Insulin	Hypoglycemia
Antidiabetic agents	Sulfonylureas	Hypoglycemia
Antidiabetic agents	Meglitinides	Hypoglycemia
Cardiovascular agents	Beta-blockers	Orthostatic hypotension, dizziness, syncope, bradycardia, impaired cerebral perfusion
Cardiovascular agents	Alpha-blockers	Orthostatic hypotension, dizziness, syncope, bradycardia, impaired cerebral perfusion
Cardiovascular agents	Calcium channel blockers	Orthostatic hypotension, dizziness, syncope, bradycardia, impaired cerebral perfusion
Cardiovascular agents	Antiarrhythmics	Orthostatic hypotension, dizziness, syncope, bradycardia, impaired cerebral perfusion
Cardiovascular agents	Diuretics	Orthostatic hypotension, dizziness, syncope, bradycardia, impaired cerebral perfusion
Cardiovascular agents	Diuretic Combinations	Orthostatic hypotension, dizziness, syncope, bradycardia, impaired cerebral perfusion
Cardiovascular agents	Central alpha2-agonists	Orthostatic hypotension, dizziness, syncope, bradycardia, impaired cerebral perfusion
Cardiovascular agents	Direct arterial vasodilators	Orthostatic hypotension, dizziness, syncope, bradycardia, impaired cerebral perfusion
Cardiovascular agents	Inotropic agents	Orthostatic hypotension, dizziness, syncope, bradycardia, impaired cerebral perfusion
Cardiovascular agents	Peripheral adrenergic antagonists	Orthostatic hypotension, dizziness, syncope, bradycardia, impaired cerebral perfusion
Psychotropic agents	Benzodiazepines	Psychomotor impairment, sedation, orthostatic hypotension, confusion, dizziness, confusion
Psychotropic agents	Hypnotics	Psychomotor impairment, sedation, orthostatic hypotension, confusion, dizziness, confusion
Psychotropic agents	Antipsychotics	Psychomotor impairment, sedation, orthostatic hypotension, confusion, dizziness, confusion
Psychotropic agents	Sedating Antidepressants	Psychomotor impairment, sedation, orthostatic hypotension, confusion, dizziness, confusion
Analgesics	Opioids	Sedation, confusion
Analgesics	morphine	Sedation, confusion
Analgesics	codeine	Sedation, confusion
Analgesics	hydrocodone	Sedation, confusion
Analgesics	oxycodone	Sedation, confusion
Analgesics	Central analgesics	Sedation, confusion
Analgesics	NSAIDs	Sedation, confusion
Anticonvulsants	phenobarbital	Sedation, psychomotor impairment, confusion
Anticholinergics	Sedating Antihistamines	Sedation, confusion
Anticholinergics	diphenhydramine	Sedation, confusion
Anticholinergics	Antimuscarinics	Sedation, confusion
Anticholinergics	Antispasmodics	Sedation, confusion
Anticholinergics	Skeletal muscle relaxants	Sedation, confusion

Data Source: University of Nebraska Medical Center, Summary
For a detailed list visit: http://www.unmc.edu/patient-safety/_documents/meds-with-fallrisk-brand-generic-table-2013.pdf

FIGURE 7.1 Medications that increase STF risk

CHAPTER 8

PETS

Over 85,000 falls treated in emergency rooms every year are caused by our pets, specifically dogs and cats. A study prepared by the Centers for Disease Control and Prevention (CDC) found that approximately 1 percent of all fall-related injuries are caused by pets.[60] Dogs are the biggest culprits, causing 88 percent of the injuries. Injuries are caused by four different scenarios: tripping or falling over the pet, walking a dog, being pushed or pulled by a dog, and tripping over a pet item or food dish.

Betti and Ed

Betti, age 75, and her husband, Ed, age 82, live in Texas. Like many retirees, they have pets, including a black Boston terrier named Sammie. Sammie likes people food. One night, Betti loaded a dinner plate high with what she describes as "piggy-portioned leftovers," from a party she'd attended the night before. She headed out onto the deck to sit on her glider and watch the sunset.

---

60   Centers for Disease Control and Prevention, "Nonfatal Fall-Related Injuries Associated with Dogs and Cats—United States, 2001–2006," *Morbidity and Mortality Weekly Report* 58, no. 11 (2009): 277–281, http://www.cdc.gov/mmwr/pdf/wk/mm5811.pdf.

"I was all ready to sit down and stuff myself when I noticed the big wooden back gate had been left open. I didn't want the dog to get out of the yard, so I got up, holding my plate so Sammie didn't eat my feast. I headed to the steps. Apparently, Sammie thought we were going somewhere with all that food. He ran under me and bam!"

Betti tripped over the dog and went airborne, falling three feet off the deck onto the concrete pavers below. Thankfully, she didn't break any bones, but she did sustain full-body bruises in a rainbow of colors. She was lucky.

"As I fell, the food exploded and the sky rained brisket, sausage, tomatoes, pasta salad, mac and cheese, cheesecake, chocolate cupcakes—I can't remember what else. I landed on my left side, still holding my empty plate. It was my good red-and-white transferware after all. Sammie cleaned up all the food.

"Two months later, I was impressed that I was able to recover from a fall like that. I felt like superwoman. Nothing was broken, and all my teeth were safe. Although I still think about that cheesecake."

She can laugh about it now, but Sammie continues to be a hazard. Six months later, Betti got up early to drive Ed to a doctor's appointment. She heard a crash, then loud cussing. It was Ed tripping over one of Sammie's toys.

There are many articles that discuss the benefits of pet ownership and most experts agree that the benefits exceed the risks. The things that you can do to prevent pet-related STF injuries fall into three categories: obedience training, location awareness and crating, and clean up.

Seek the advice of a good trainer to help teach your dog good leash manners and walking behaviors. Your dog or puppy should be taught not to pull, not to lunge at other dogs or people, and not to wander around you or cut in front of you. Training your pup to stay or sit will help keep her from getting under foot.

Be aware of your pet's location. This is especially important at night and in poorly lit hallways. Use nightlights and glow-in-the-dark pet collars to help you keep track of your dog or cat. When performing activities that prevent you from tracking your pet's location, like unloading the car, crate your pet or put her in another room so that she doesn't get underfoot. If your dog rushes down the stairs when the doorbell rings, let her go first so you won't get bumped or pushed on the stairway.

Clean up after your pet. I've spent many hours picking up after my kids, and cleaning up after my dogs is more work. Get a basket or box for your pet's toys. While you can't control where the toys end up, you can move them out of your walking path when your dog isn't chewing or playing. Keep food and water bowls out of main walkways and, if your pet is a messy eater or sloppy drinker, clean up after her frequently.

CHAPTER 9

DISTRACTED WALKING

According to the National Safety Council (NSC), distracted walking caused around two thousand emergency room visits in 2011. We live in an age when our attention is pulled in many different directions. We try to multitask at every opportunity. This sets the perfect stage for STF injuries caused by distractions. Distractions contribute to fall injuries in many different ways, but distracted walking seems to be a rising cause for concern. Cell phones are the primary culprit, but distractions can come in other forms, such as an intense conversation with your walking companion or simply looking at something more interesting that the path in front of you.

Distracted driving has been an area of interest for the National Highway Traffic Safety Association for years. The NSC estimates that 26 percent of all traffic crashes are associated with drivers distracted by using cell phones.[61] So it should come as no surprise, with the rise in cell phone usage, that distracted walking is a growing problem. In 2015, the NSC added distracted walking statistics to its Injury Facts Report:[62]

---

61   National Safety Council, Annual Estimate of Cell Phone Crashes 2013, http://www.nsc.org/DistractedDrivingDocuments/CPK/Attributable-Risk-Summary.pdf.

62   National Safety Council, *Injury Facts*, 2015 edition, 153, http://www.nsc.org/Membership%20Site%20Document%20Library/2015%20Injury%20Facts/NSC_InjuryFacts2015Ed.pdf.

- 74 percent of the injuries were related to cell phone usage (12 percent while texting, 62 percent while talking)
- 80 percent were from falls
- 52 percent occurred at home
- 54 percent happened to people age 40 or younger
- 68 percent happened to females

Fort Lee, New Jersey

Officials in Fort Lee, New Jersey, decided that awareness campaigns weren't quite doing the trick, so they've passed a city ban on texting while jaywalking.[63] Tickets will be issued for "dangerous walking," which includes texting and walking. The idea is to address the point of the walker's commute where they're most at risk for being hit by a car. State legislatures in New Jersey, New York, Illinois, Arkansas, Nevada, and Hawaii have considered similar statewide bans, but as of this writing, none have passed into law.[64]

Texting not only takes your eyes off the sidewalk, but also slows your speed, affects your gait, and disrupts your ability to walk in a straight line, according to a study published in 2014.[65] Pedestrians who text while walking can stray into traffic, sometimes with deadly consequences, or trip over bumps in the sidewalk. The study also found that texting pedestrians tend to walk more stiffly, which made them more likely to fall when they encounter an obstacle because their posture makes it harder for them to catch themselves.

63   Chenda Ngak, "Texting While Walking Banned in NJ Town," *CBS News*, May 15, 2012, http://www.cbsnews.com/news/texting-while-walking-banned-in-nj-town/.

64   Chris Matyszczyk, "Will This State Ban Texting While Walking?" *CNET*, March 27, 2016, http://www.cnet.com/news/state-politician-moves-to-ban-texting-while-walking/.

65   Siobhan Schabrun, et al., "Texting and Walking: Strategies for Postural Control and Implications for Safety," *PLOS ONE*, January 22, 2014, doi: 10.1371/journal.pone.0084312.

Prevention

There's a large disparity between the number of people who believe that distracted walking is a problem and those who admit to being part of the problem. A study conducted by the American Academy of Orthopaedic Surgeons found that 78 percent of US adults believe that distracted walking is a "serious" issue; however, 74 percent say "other people" are usually or always walking while distracted, while only 29 percent say the same about themselves.[66] If the blame is always on the other guy, we won't make changes in our own behavior to improve the situation. Prevention must start with you. If you text and walk, you're part of the problem and you're at a higher risk for an STF injury. The next step is self-discipline; put down the phone and pay attention to where you're walking.

Any call, text, or other distraction needs to be managed. Make a decision to either stop walking and take that call or defer the call until you can give it your full attention. Make getting to your destination your top priority and stay focused on the task at hand.

---

66   American Academy of Orthopaedic Surgeons, "Distracted Walking: A Serious Issue for You, Not Me," *Science Daily,* December 2, 2015, www.sciencedaily.com/releases/2015/12/151202132710.htm.

CHAPTER 10

OTHER CAUSES OF FALLS

This chapter covers other common causes of falls that haven't been previously discussed. Because every home is unique, I encourage you to refer to Chapter 25, "Home Audit Checklist," for a walking guide to help you identify specific hazards where you live.

Furniture

Think of the placement of your furniture as a sort of skeleton inside your home. While a chair or couch encroaching into a main walkway poses a problem in itself, the way your chairs, tables, couches, and other furnishings are positioned can also play a role in where items get left on the floor.

For example, when you sit in a particular chair you may take off your shoes there. If the chair is in a pathway in your home, those shoes may pose a tripping hazard. Establish patterns and habits that help you avoid creating trip hazards.

Electric cords

Look at the way electrical cords run in your house. In some cases, you may need to get creative about how you run those cords, like attaching them to the wall at the baseboard to keep them out of the way. There are also cord protectors that can be laid across walkways and keep the cord close to the ground. You could also have an electrician install additional outlets where needed.

This is also a problem if you temporarily need electricity in a location for a special project. Running an extension cord so you can use power tools is normal. However, you need to tape that cord down to the floor or clearly mark the cord as a danger. Never leave the extension cord in place when you leave your work area. I realize that it may be a lot of work to pick up your extension cord when you stop for lunch but not doing it is like setting a trap for other people who may wander by. Rather than having to apologize to your daughter or your wife for sending them to the emergency room, take an extra minute and avoid that risk. If you use extension cords regularly invest in a cord protector.

Area rugs and throw rugs

Rugs pose two different types of hazards: the first is when you trip on an edge of the rug, and the second is when the rug itself slips when you step on it. If you notice either of these problems, remove, replace, or secure the rug. Watch for the small slips and trips that occur here. Any small slip or trip means you have a problem that needs attention. Don't blame yourself for being clumsy or expect your athletic ability to save you in the future. You're denying the inevitable.

Secure rugs to the floor using double-sided tape or a secure underlay. Get rid of mats that are fraying or curling at the edges—there's no way to fix them. Watch for rugs that have too much of a height differential. If it causes you to stumble just once, get rid of it. The next stumble may result in a serious injury.

Clutter

There's natural clutter, like leaves, and there's man-made (or child-made) clutter, like toys and tools that are left on the walkways and stairs. Clutter in your path should serve as a warning to tread carefully. Clutter by itself isn't usually the cause of a fall. Clutter by itself is easy to spot and avoid. Clutter becomes a problem when it's combined with other factors like hiding uneven sidewalks and pathways, distractions that cause us to pay less attention to our walking path, and poor lighting.

Watch where you're walking, walk *around*—not over or through—clutter when you can, and, more importantly, keep pathways clear. Don't count on your physical skills to save you when you walk on slippery surfaces. Pay special attention to walkways that are used in low light. A great example is keeping that path to the bathroom clear, just in case you have to make a middle of the night journey.

Do you do this? Sometimes I create dangerous clutter. If I have something that I want to take upstairs, but I don't want to make a special trip, I'll place it on the first or second stair so I remember to take it with me the next time I go that way. Then something happens and I run upstairs in a hurry and don't take my item. This now has become a potential fall hazard. If you use this memory trick be sure to place the item clearly out of the walking path and off the stairs so you won't risk tripping on it.

Provide a place for everything and make sure that everything is in its place. Toy boxes, shoe cubbies, and shelves can help keep things off the floor and make your home safer.

Wet conditions

Wet conditions increase the likelihood of a slip. Spills are an obvious problem, but don't just think about spills on the floor—spills on a table or counter will travel to the floor if they're not cleaned up promptly. Rain, puddles, and mud also create higher-risk situations. The danger increases when the wet is mixed with other factors, like freezing or near freezing temperatures; ground cover, like leaves or debris; or mold and mildew that may have grown because of continuous damp situations.

Clean up any spills immediately. If you can't clean it up, walk around the area. If you must walk through a wet area, expect the area to be slippery. Use caution when walking on any wet area.

Good housekeeping

Much of what we've been talking about is simply good housekeeping. To prevent slips, clean up spills immediately. If you've mopped the floor, make others in the house aware that it could be slippery. Pick up trash clutter that may interfere with your walkway as soon as you spot them.

Aside from teaching yourself new habits of placing items out of the walkway, you may also need to teach these habits to everyone in your household. The actions you take today will help to save you from a fall injury in the future.

SECTION TWO

Where We Fall

The first section discussed the conditions that create fall hazards and the circumstances that will increase our risk of a STF injury. This section focuses in on the locations where most STF injuries occur. Sometimes it is difficult to separate the why we fall from the where we fall. When this occurred I made a judgment call and placed that topic in what I thought was the best section.

The chapters in this section are loosely listed in order of most frequent cause of STF injury. I say loosely because, at the time of this writing, there are no comprehensive studies that rank the causes of falls by location. Capturing this type of data becomes challenging because a STF injury might have multiple contributing causes. For example, a STF injury may have occurred on stairs, in poorly lit conditions. So would the cause for this STF injury be classified as stairway or lighting? You get the picture. Whenever possible I quote numbers from individual research studies to demonstrate the general magnitude of the problem in a particular 'where' but these frequency numbers are not directly comparable because they will have different timeframes or data sources.

Stairs and handrails are the most frequent location for STF injuries generating over one million STF injuries or approximately 15 percent of all emergency room visits caused by falls. Ladders and step stools cause the most severe injuries because of the impact from a fall from height. Our bathrooms, kitchens, and hallways have conditions that increase our risks associated with STF injuries. The purpose of this section is to highlight those conditions so you can avoid or prevent future injuries.

The majority of people who have fallen have done so in a place they already recognized as a STF risk. Once they fall, they often say if only I'd fixed that problem when I first noticed it I would not have to deal with this injury now. You already know exactly where the most dangerous part of your home is because you've tripped, slipped, or fallen there before. You now need to fix that problem before it becomes an injury.

Factoid #6

Deaths Caused Falls Mapped by State Show Some Surprises

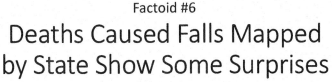

States Ranked by Number of Deaths Caused by Falls per 100K of Population

For Years: 2008-2010

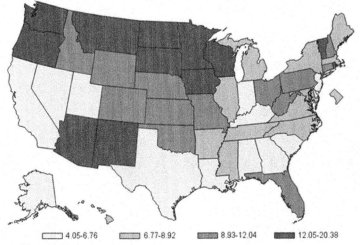

4.05-6.76	6.77-8.92	8.93-12.04	12.05-20.38

Map Produced by: The Statistics, Programming & Economics Branch, National Center of Injury Prevention & Control, CDC
Data Sources: NCES National Vital Statistics System for numbers of deaths; US Census Bureau for Population

- Alaska is one of the safest states.
- Arizona and New Mexico are shown to be amongst the most dangerous.
- We do not understand why:
  - Michigan is much safer than Wisconsin,
  - Vermont is much safer than Maine
  - Ohio, Pennsylvania and West Virginia are more dangerous than New Jersey and Indiana

The Work Environment is Much Safer from Fall Injuries and Deaths

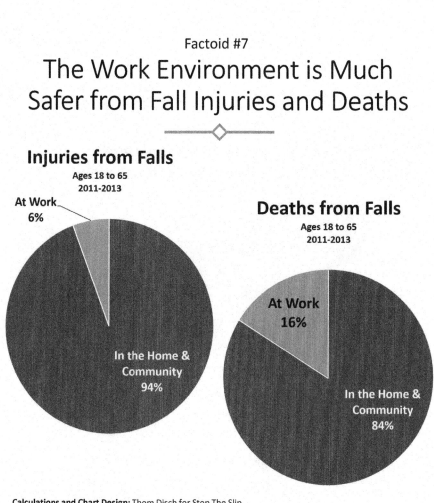

Injuries from Falls
Ages 18 to 65
2011-2013

At Work
6%

In the Home & Community
94%

Deaths from Falls
Ages 18 to 65
2011-2013

At Work
16%

In the Home & Community
84%

Calculations and Chart Design: Thom Disch for <u>Stop The Slip</u>
Data Source: Bureau of Labor Statistics; and NEISS All Injury Program operated by the
Consumer Product Safety Commission (CPSC).
National Center for Injury Prevention and Control, CDC using WISQARS™.

- Falls cause more accidents away from your workplace.
- You need to implement slip. Trip and fall prevention actions that are similar to the policies implemented at most businesses.
- This analysis is limited to individuals of working age (18 to 65), thus excluding any bias from seniors and children.

Factoid #8

Risk of Fall Injury by Industry

◇

Number of Fall Injuries Per 10K Employees
Annual 2013

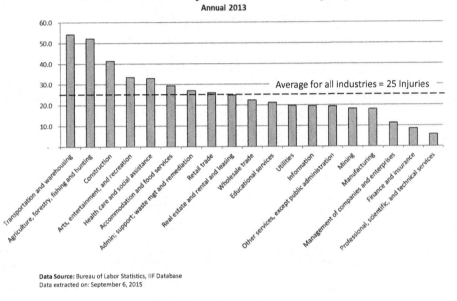

Data Source: Bureau of Labor Statistics, IIF Database
Data extracted on: September 6, 2015

- Work environment is one of the leading determinants of fall risk in the work place.
- Mining and Manufacturing are amongst the safest industries for falls.
- Arts, entertainment and recreation and Healthcare and social assistance are amongst the most dangerous industries for falls

Factoid #9

Most Fall Injuries Occur
on the Same Level

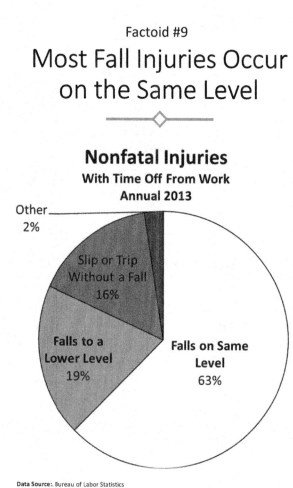

Nonfatal Injuries
With Time Off From Work
Annual 2013

Other
2%

Slip or Trip
Without a Fall
16%

Falls to a
Lower Level
19%

Falls on Same
Level
63%

Data Source:. Bureau of Labor Statistics
Data extracted on: September 6, 2015 (11:47:41 AM)

- This data is only available for injuries that happen at work.
- Falling when climbing up stairs is considered a Fall on same level.
- Falling down the stairs is considered a Fall to a lower level.
- Injuries from slips or trips without a fall was a surprising 16%

Tubs And Showers Are The Location For Over 2/3rds Of Injuries In Bathrooms

Location of Injuries in Bathrooms

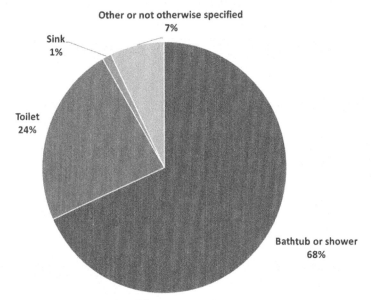

People over 14 years old
Calendar 2008

Data Source: Centers for Disease Control and Prevention, Morbidity and Mortality Weekly Report; June 10, 2011 / 60(22);729-733, Nonfatal Bathroom Injuries Among Persons Aged ≥15 Years

- Over 200,000 ER visits per year are from injuries in the bathroom.
- Falls cause over 80% of all injuries in the bathroom.
- Getting out of the bathtub is the leading cause of bathroom injuries.
- 64% of bathroom injuries happen to women.

CHAPTER 11

STAIRS AND HANDRAILS

In 2013, according to the US Consumer Product Safety Commission, emergency rooms treated over 1.3 million injuries that occurred on stairs or in conjunction with handrails or banisters.[67] That represents 4 percent of all emergency room visits and 15 percent of fall-related injuries. This category is complicated because there are so many different types of steps and many different ways that people can be injured on them. For example, people not only fall down stairs, they fall up them. (I can personally attest to this. It usually happens when I'm in a hurry and I miss my footing.) A study performed by Templer, Archea, and Cohen determined that 8 percent of injuries happen when going up the stairs and 92 percent happen when going down.[68] I was surprised that the falling up number was so high, but it makes me feel a little less clumsy.

Clearly stairs can be dangerous, but we use them every day and, most of the time, without incident. So when do stairs become dangerous? There may be a single step or there can be an entire staircase. The design varies from indoor

---

67   National Safety Council, *Injury Facts,* 2015 edition; U.S. Consumer Product Safety Commission, National Electronic Injury Surveillance System (NEISS), 168, http://www.nsc.org/Membership%20Site%20Document%20Library/2015%20Injury%20Facts/NSC_InjuryFacts2015Ed.pdf.

68   John Templer, et al., "Study of Factors Associated with Risk of Work-Related Stairway Falls," *Journal of Safety Research* 16, no. 4 (1985): 183–196, doi: 10.1016/0022-4375(85)90005-2.

to outdoor, from simple to architecturally elegant. Stairs can be made of basic lumber or finished hardwood, metal or concrete, carpeted or polished stone, or tile. So, with all this variety, how do we address the number of fall injuries related to stairs?

Becky and Ed

Becky and Ed live with their children in a charming Victorian-style home with hardwood floors. The house is well maintained, but it was built in the 1950s and, like many older homes, it's drafty. To help keep the floors clean, shoes aren't allowed to be worn indoors; the family enters the house through the mudroom and stores their shoes in cubbies when they take them off.

Today is Becky's fiftieth birthday. Ed, who hit that milestone six years ago, gets up early to make her coffee and breakfast in bed. It's a particularly cold February morning, and Ed puts on the socks he wore last night, knowing that tile floor in the kitchen will be cold. He comes out the bedroom and starts down the hardwood stairs and then it happens: his foot slips out from under him and he falls all the way down the steps on his back.

If you've ever gone up or down a hardwood staircase in your stocking feet, you know how risky this situation can be. You can go up and down the stairs safely a hundred times, but on the hundred and first time you feel your foot slip—not a lot, but enough to make you think, wow, I've got to be more careful, one of these days I'm going to kill myself on these steps. Not two minutes later, you've forgotten the entire thing and you go about your day—until the next time you and your stocking feet slip.

Here are two safer alternatives: buy yourself a pair of warm slippers with good non-slip sole, or install an STF prevention product on your stairs and in other areas where the hardwood floors put you at risk for a slip, trip, or fall.

Because slips and fall on stairs is such a complex category, I've broken the prevention category down into two sections: unsafe acts and unsafe conditions.

Prevention for unsafe acts

As the name implies, unsafe acts are actions that we take increasing our risk of an injury. Conventional safety management says that about 90 percent of all injuries are caused by unsafe acts. Fixing this type of problem requires us to first recognize the unsafe act and then to change our behavior. In most situations, once you've recognized the risky behavior, the change to a safer action is obvious. Some of the most common unsafe acts on stairways include:

- **Failure to use a handrail:** Handrails provide an extra point of stability. When using stairs without a handrail, we'll often have only a single foot, a single point of contact, on the stairs. Using a handrail increases stability and provides a way to recover should we start to fall. Many businesses have found this to be so important they mandate the use of handrails in their safety manuals. Always use a handrail when using the stairs.

- **Faulty or unsafe footwear:** This includes worn out shoes, slippery soles, high heels, clothing that falls below foot level, untied shoelaces, and stocking feet. We've all experienced just how slippery stocking feet can be on hardwood floors and stairs, yet we perform this unsafe act because wearing socks is a simple solution to cold feet. Changing your behavior can make you safer. If you have hardwood floors in your home, buy a nice pair of warm slippers with a nonslip sole or cover the stairs with a carpet runner or apply a nonslip tread to the stair (visit PeopleTreads.com for one option).

- **Inattention or distractions:** Not paying attention when walking up and down stairs is dangerous (see Chapter 9, "Distracted Walking," for an in-depth discussion of this topic).

- **Carrying children or objects:** Carrying anything on the stairs increases your risk of an STF accident. Here are some of the reasons that you're more likely to be injured when carrying something on the stairs:
  - Your attention is split between what you're holding and walking on the stairs.
  - You've changed your weight distribution and balance.

- A greater physical effort is required and this can result in muscle failure.
- Your hands aren't available to hold onto the handrails.
- Your view of the stairs may be blocked by the object you're carrying.

Carrying children down stairs alone results in five thousand child injuries a year.[69] This is the number one cause of child–stair injuries after you exclude children who fell without mention of another action or object. It's interesting to note that children who are injured when being carried are more severely injured than those who fall on their own.

If you have to carry something on the stairs, manage the load. Focus on carrying things safely on the stairs. For example, making multiple trips with smaller and lighter loads will make you safer.

- **Spills or clutter:** Keep your stairs clean and clear of clutter. Clean up spills immediately. If something is dropped or left on the stairs, move it to a safe location. Don't plan on doing it later or walking around the problem; fix it when you see it.
- **Missed footing:** Pay attention to walking safely on stairs. Make sure your foot is solidly on each stair before taking your next step.
- Hurrying: Oftentimes we're focused on the many things on our to-do-lists. Rushing to get to the next task is a form of distraction. Take a breath, slow down, and focus on the task at hand: walking safely on the stairs.

Prevention for unsafe conditions

Unsafe conditions include stairs and handrails that are missing, poorly designed or in need of repair. These are situations that can result in a lawsuit. A standard step has a 7-inch rise with an 11-inch-wide tread. We expect this—our muscle memory is trained for this pattern. Variation from this standard increases the likelihood of an STF injury.

---

69   Ashley Zielinski, et al., "Stair-Related Injuries to Young Children Treated in US Emergency Departments 1999–2008," *Pediatrics* 129, no. 4 (2012): 721–727, doi: 10.1542/peds.2011-2314.

Unsafe conditions usually require a cash investment to fix whatever is broken or out of compliance. Of course, that's easier to do when it's your property or when the fix is inexpensive. What do you do when it isn't your property or the cost exceeds your budget? You must adjust your behavior. Slow down, be extra cautious, avoid all distractions, and watch where you place your feet. Sometimes it even makes sense to take a different path.

Here are some common unsafe stair conditions and recommendations for making them safer:

- **Weather:** This includes rain, snow, frost, and even mold and mildew. Porches and deck steps are common danger spots. Special treatment for slippery stairs includes applying a nonslip product (visit Handitreads.com for one option).
- **Loose, missing, or inadequate handrails:** As mentioned earlier, handrails provide extra security and should be used whenever possible. Make sure that handrails are available and secure. This is also true for locations with just one or two steps, like a transition between your home and garage.
- **Broken steps and stairways:** If you notice a stair that needs to be repaired, take care of it right away. Common problems include loose, unlevel, cracked, or broken steps; broken or chipped stair edges; and nosings (front-edge guards) which are bent and do not lie flat.
- **Design flaws:** The worst design flaw occurs when stair riser height varies on the same set of stairs. Research has shown that we typically see only the first and last three steps; we negotiate the rest of the stairway without looking.[70] This means that when riser height varies, we're taken by surprise and our balance is affected. Stairs that have a rise greater than 7 3/4 inches will cause us to stumble. A rise of less than 6 inches will require a lot of extra steps and will feel unnatural. Stair treads that are too narrow provide too little space to properly place our feet. Treads that are too wide often create an unnatural gait, and require extra concentration to keep from landing on the stair edge.

---

70   Wayne Maynard and George Brogmus, "Reducing Slips, Trips, and Falls in Stairways," *EHS Today,* October 1, 2007, http://ehstoday.com/ppe/fall-protection/ehs_imp_75425.

CHAPTER 12

LADDERS AND STEP STOOLS

According to the Bureau of Labor Statistics (BLS), we're three times more likely to be injured on a level surface than in a fall from an elevation.[71] However, it should come as no surprise that a fall from an elevation causes more serious injuries than a fall on a level walking surface.

Step stools and ladders are great tools for making us safer, but that's true only if they're used correctly. Here's a common situation: It's the holidays. You want to get the serving platter down from the top shelf. You can't reach the top shelf without assistance. Do you grab the kitchen chair that's right at your fingertips and step up to the platter? Or do you spend the time to locate the step stool (if you even own one) and safely bring the platter down? We all know the right thing to do, but finding that step stool, positioning it, and returning it to its proper place is a lot more work. Most people just use the kitchen chair.

The next time you reach for that chair, think about the following:

- The height of a chair makes it dangerous to be used as a step stool. The seating area, or as it's being used here, the stepping elevation, on a typical chair is approximately 20 inches high. That's close to the

---

71   United States Department of Labor, Bureau of Labor Statistics, "Injuries, Illnesses, and Fatalities," 2015, http://www.bls.gov/iif/.

height of three steps on a stairway. Stepping up or stepping down the height of three steps is challenging for even the most athletic of us. A step stool has steps that are in the eight- to eleven-inch height range.

- The seating area of the chair isn't designed for foot traffic. Your derriere spreads your weight out more evenly than a single foot. Some chair seats will not support the concentrated weight of a single foot. The chair seat may be cushioned, which makes it difficult to step on. If it doesn't have a cushion, it may be slippery.

- Once you've retrieved the platter from the upper shelf, you'll have to take a single step down twenty inches holding onto it. This means that your balance will be further compromised and that increases your risk of falling. Also keep in mind that if you fall, you'll drop the platter.

- It may seem obvious, but because it's the common cause of falls, I have to mention it: never climb on a chair with wheels. Wheels on a chair make it more difficult to get on the chair and, once you're on it, the chair can roll out from under you.

- As I've said many times, falls are the number one reason people go to the emergency room.[72] You may save some time using a chair as a step stool if you can do it successfully, but if you make a mistake the amount of time you'll spend getting treatment for your injury and recovering will far exceed the amount of time you would have saved.

Ladders are step stools on steroids. They let us extend our reach even further, but they also require much greater care and safety when being used. According to the National Institute for Occupational Safety and Health (NIOSH), more than 500,000 Americans are treated—and about three hundred die—each year with ladder-related injuries.[73] There are two basic types of ladders: stepladders, that stand on their own and form an "A" shape when set up, and extension ladders, which rest against a wall or a building.

---

72 Centers for Disease Control and Prevention, "National Estimates of the 10 Leading Causes of Nonfatal Injuries Treated in Hospital Emergency Departments, United States, 2013," http://www.cdc.gov/injury/images/lc-charts/leading_cause_of_nonfatal_injury_2013-a.gif.

73 National Institute for Occupational Safety and Health, "NIOSH Ladder Safety App," http://www.cdc.gov/niosh/topics/falls/mobileapp.html

The number one cause of ladder injuries is incorrect ladder set up. This causes approximately 40 percent of all ladder-related injuries.[74] Other causes for injury include not choosing the right ladder for the right job; poor ladder maintenance, including using broken or damaged ladders; and user error, which includes things like overreaching, improper carrying of objects up a ladder, and missteps while on the ladder.

Bob and Ashley

Ashley remembers the day well. It was a beautiful Saturday, the perfect start to summer in Chicago, where she'd been living for two years. She made the trip home to see her parents at least once a month and she was planning on being home on Monday.

That afternoon, her mom called and told her that her dad, Bob, had fallen off a ladder and twisted his ankle. Bob was heading out to mow the lawn when he noticed that the gutter along the driveway was overflowing with leaves. So, like many homeowners, he decided to take care of it himself. He got out the extension ladder and set it up on the driveway like he'd done dozens of times before.

Bob started climbing up the ladder and wasn't more than about four feet off the ground when it happened. Anyone who's used an extension ladder has felt it: that sense of helplessness when you're off the ground and you feel the base of ladder move. Normally, it moves only a fraction of an inch and then settles back down—but not this time. Bob wasn't sure if he set the foot of the ladder on a pebble or if one of the rubber feet wasn't set level on the ground. Maybe he set up the ladder at just a little too much of an angle. Whatever the cause, the ladder slid backward away from the house. Bob was faced with two choices, neither of them good: he could hold on for dear life and crash to the ground with the ladder, or he could jump off and hope for the best. He chose to jump.

Bob landed feet first and felt the pain in his left foot. His neighbor, who had seen the whole thing, rushed over to make sure Bob was all right. He

---

74   Ibid.

helped Bob hobble into the house and, after some gentle chiding from his wife, he settled into his favorite chair with his ankle propped up.

It's often difficult to determine if a foot is broken. In Bob's case, there were no protruding bones, no torn or broken skin, and no obvious deformity. So Bob took a wait-and-see attitude instead of going to the emergency room. By Sunday, the swelling was worse and his entire foot was covered in colorful bruises. Still, he thought, how bad could it be? And Ashley was coming home on Monday—if it wasn't better by then, Ashley could take him to his regular doctor.

On Monday morning, Bob, who worked as a courier for the local hospital system, reached out to some of his connections. The pain continued to get worse and the swelling wasn't going down. By the time Ashley came home, Bob had an appointment at the local orthopedic center. The doctor examined the foot and took x-rays, which showed that Bob had fractured his heel bone. (This type of fracture is sometimes called a fireman's break, because it's often seen in firefighters when they fall through a floor.) The doctor sent Bob and Ashley to a nearby emergency room. At the emergency room, where the diagnosis was confirmed and Bob's very swollen foot was put into a soft cast. No further action could be taken due to the swelling, so Bob was sent home with pain medication and anti-inflammatories and strict instructions to rest and keep off the injured foot.

Bob rested and waited. After several subsequent doctor visits, it was decided that Bob required surgery. But the surgery would have to wait until the swelling went down. It took six weeks for the swelling to subside. When the surgery was finally performed, it took twenty-six screws and bracing hardware to secure the break.

Bob's next challenge came when his surgical cut became infected. It was now late August and the first efforts were to treat this with antibiotics. It soon became clear that additional surgeries were required. Three additional surgeries were performed over a one-week period to clean up the infection. Then it was a matter of waiting. There was serious concern as to whether the surgical cut would heal. If it didn't heal properly, the only other option would be to amputate the foot.

Falls can produce injuries that lead to unforeseen complications. Those complications can result in very serious health consequences or even death. In Bob's case, patience and rest finally paid off: eight months after his fall, Bob was able to finally take his first unaided step. He still has a ways to go with rehab and he had to take early retirement, but his future looks bright.

Prevention

The simplest thing is to keep frequently used items within easy reach so you won't need to climb up to get them. Then whenever you need to reach for something, use a step stool or ladder. Don't climb on a chair or other object not designed for the job. You may think you're saving time and effort, but you're putting your health at risk every time you take that shortcut. The National Safety Council provides some great safety tips[75] and The National Institute for Occupational Safety and Health (NIOSH) even has a ladder safety app that you can download to your smartphone.[76] The app includes topics like how to choose a ladder; an inspection guide for making sure your ladder is safe to use; how to set up your ladder, including a measuring tool to verify that it's set up at a safe angle; how to safely use your ladder; and a list of accessories you can use to make sure your ladder is safe and secure. The following list of preventive steps draws heavily on the information provided in the app:

Choose the right ladder

- Think about the needs for the task at hand.
- Choose the right size and style.
- Follow the directions on the ladder before you climb.
- Answer these questions: How high do you need to reach? Are you working against a wall or other support? How much weight will the ladder need to hold? Is it an indoor or outdoor job?

75 National Safety Council, "Take Ladder Safety One Rung at a Time," http://www.nsc.org/ Membership%20Site%20Document%20Library/E-Newsletter-Content/ST-Ladder-Safety.pdf.

76 National Institute for Occupational Safety and Health, "NIOSH Ladder Safety App," http://www.cdc.gov/niosh/topics/falls/mobileapp.html.

Set up your ladder properly

- Always put it on a firm, solid base. If you must put the ladder on a soft surface, place a board under the ladder's feet.
- Set up your ladder at the proper angle. A straight or extension ladder should be placed one foot away from the surface it's resting on for every four feet of the ladder's height.
- Never lean a straight or extension ladder against a windowpane or other unstable surface.
- Securely fasten straight or extension ladders to an upper support so they're unlikely to slip or tilt to one side.
- Make sure stepladders are open completely before climbing.
- Guard doorways and walkways near your ladder. Remember even the slightest bump can cause you to lose your balance and fall.
- Never place a ladder on another object to gain additional height; instead, use a longer ladder.

Follow these safe use guidelines

- Face the ladder and always grip the rungs, not the side rails.
- Always keep three points of contact with the ladder: two hands and one foot or two feet and one hand.
- Never get off a ladder from the side.
- Make sure extension ladders extend three feet above the roof or platform you're trying to reach.
- Don't stand higher than the third rung from the top.
- Don't lean or overreach; reposition the ladder instead.
- Don't climb while carrying tools; use a tool belt.
- Wear slip-resistant shoes.
- Never let someone climb up to bring you something; only one person should be on a ladder at a time.

Be mindful of these additional safety considerations

- Inspect the ladder for damage before each use.
- Don't use extension ladders in windy or inclement weather. If bad weather arises, climb down immediately and wait for it to pass.
- Clean the ladder after each use to prevent dirt buildup, especially if it's left outside in wet or muddy conditions.

Consult the following websites for additional ladder safety tips

US Consumer Product Safety Commission, Ladder Safety 101

cpsc.gov/onsafety/2011/12/ladder-safety-101/

Occupational Safety and Health Administration, Falling Off Ladders Can Kill

osha.gov/Publications/OSHA3625.pdf

American Ladder Institute

americanladderinstitute.org/

CHAPTER 13

POOR LIGHTING AND REDUCED VISION

I recently moved into a new house. The first few nights after we moved in were incredibly dangerous. Learning to navigate new paths and stair locations was especially challenging when the sun went down. For me, the most important path was the one to the bathroom. I felt guilty about waking up in the middle of the night and waking up my wife by turning on the lights so I could find a safe pathway to relief. New furniture locations and surprise sleeping spots for our pets increased my risk of an STF injury. It didn't take long before I was at the local hardware store buying nightlights, which I placed at the top and bottom of each stairway. I also made sure I could see the paths that might be walked after the lights went out. This helped so much that I now pack a couple of nightlights in my luggage when I'm traveling and want to be a little bit safer in my hotel room.

As we age, our vision declines.[77] This could be for a variety of reasons, ranging from part of the natural aging process to poor nutrition to a medical condition such as diabetes or cataracts. Many people notice these changes

---

77   US Department of Health and Human Services, National Institutes of Health, "Your Aging Eyes: How You See as Time Goes By," *NIH News in Health*, January 2011, https://newsinhealth.nih.gov/issue/jan2011/feature1.

beginning to happen as early as age 35. The result is often reading glasses or progressive lenses, as well as slower reaction to changes in light and even night blindness.

David Pu'u

We've already discussed how stairs present a slip-and-trip hazard of their own, but adding darkness to climbing stairs while running is a recipe for disaster. David Pu'u, an international photographer and cinematographer, learned this the hard way. While his job requires him to be physically fit and involves walking on surfaces that present many different STF hazards, like seaweed-slippery rocks and uneven cobblestoned streets, the big fall he remembers happened inside an apartment building where he and his wife were staying.

"We had booked a fantastic place to stay in a high-rise near a great beach in Portugal," he recalled. "Our big apartment was on the thirteenth floor—I know, not a good omen—and it was serviced by a very old elevator system. It had a broad, well laid-out stairwell lit by automatic (motion sensor activated) lights.

"I needed a workout so I did what I've done many times before: I ran up and down the sixteen floors of stairs a few times. As I started down from the thirteenth floor, all was good. I was slowly and steadily beginning to warm up," he said.

Four floors later, the man who navigates stormy oceans and seafoam-covered rocks without a hitch found himself falling into darkness. He tumbled down the steps and wound up in a crumpled heap on the concrete landing of the ninth floor, the victim of a fall resulting from a sudden onset of poor eyesight caused by darkness.

When what we're seeing changes faster than our mind, there's a sort of hiccup in our eyesight. This hiccup doesn't pose a problem—unless you're involved in a critical, second-by-second event (like Pu'u was), where timing is split-second dependent. So, as he began to run down the stairs in the dark, he triggered the motion sensors in the stairwell, but by the time the lights had come up completely, he was moving to the next floor, from light to dark to light to dark. This is the same experience you have when crossing from a well-lit space into a dark one. It takes a few seconds for your eyes to adjust. Chances are if the stairwell lighting hadn't been motion activated, Pu'u wouldn't have fallen. If you find yourself in a dark stairwell, make sure you use the handrail and take each step carefully and slowly.

Prevention

Low vision and poor lighting can combine to increase the risk of an STF injury. You can reduce your risk of falling by integrating these tips into your everyday routine:

- **Increase the amount of lighting:** With age, the muscles that control our pupils weaken. As a result, by the time we're in our sixties, we need three times more light to read than when we were in our twenties.[78] This also affects our ability to see where we're walking. More lighting means a safer pathway.
- **Install nightlights:** When we first wake up, we're naturally groggy and darkness adds to the challenge. Strategically placing nightlights throughout your home will help you avoid those hidden trip hazards.
- **Don't wear bifocal or progressive lenses when you walk, especially on stairs.** These lenses are designed for convenience, you can use a single pair of glasses to read when you are looking down at text and see at a distance when you look up. Unfortunately, the part of the lens you use to read text may be the same part you use when you're looking down at a walking path or stair treads. That means your view of your stairs will be blurry. Talk with your vision care professional about the best way to manage this problem.
- **Get proper vision care and eye exams:** In addition to providing you with crystal clear vision, your eye care professional can diagnose any eye disorders that may be affecting you. Early diagnosis and treatment is essential in keeping your vision healthy throughout your lifetime.

---

78   Ibid.

- **Use high contrast as a warning for STF risk areas:** A *New York Times* article on falls includes three short videos that show how visual impairments affect our ability to see clearly.[79] Adding high-contrast warning strips makes it much easier to see STF hazards, even if your vision is affected by low vision.

79   Katie Hafner, "Bracing for the Falls of an Aging Nation," *New York Times*, October 30, 2014, http://www.nytimes.com/interactive/2014/11/03/health/bracing-for-the-falls-of-an-aging-nation. html?_r=0.

CHAPTER 14

BATHROOMS

One of the most dangerous rooms in the home is the bathroom. Bathrooms contain a unique combination of STF hazards. Water and other slippery liquids like soap and conditioners are being used on slippery surfaces like tile and natural stone. We then add tripping hazards like bathtubs and towels all in a small confined space, it is no surprise that bathroom injuries result in over two hundred thousand emergency room visits a year.[80] Over 80 percent of those were caused by falls.

Over two-thirds of all bathroom injuries happen around the bathtub or shower. Extra caution should be used when exiting the shower because you are 4 times more likely to be injured when getting out of the shower than getting in.[81]

---

80   Centers for Disease Control and Prevention, "Nonfatal Bathroom Injuries Among Persons Aged ≥15 Years, United States, 2008," *Morbidity and Mortality Weekly Report* 60, no. 22 (2011): 729–733, http://www.cdc.gov/mmwr/preview/mmwrhtml/mm6022a1.htm.

81   Ibid.

Location of Injuries in Bathrooms

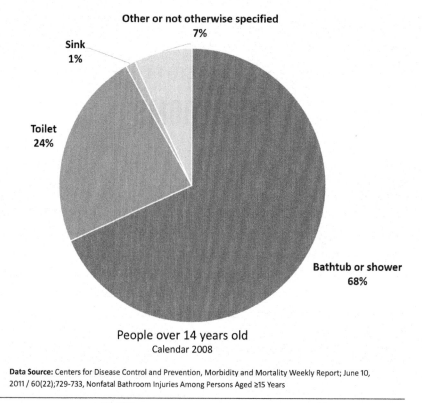

People over 14 years old
Calendar 2008

Data Source: Centers for Disease Control and Prevention, Morbidity and Mortality Weekly Report; June 10, 2011 / 60(22);729-733, Nonfatal Bathroom Injuries Among Persons Aged ≥15 Years

FIGURE 14.1 Locations of Injuries in bathrooms for adults, 2008

What is surprising is that the number emergency room visits as a result of bathroom injuries is 72 percent higher for women than for men.[82] The Centers for Disease Control (CDC) suggests that it might be physiological or it could be that women spend more time in the bathroom or it may be that men may be less likely to go to the emergency room for an injury. The actual reason for this disparity is unknown, but it is worth noting so that women are aware of

82   Ibid.

their higher STF injury rate and as a result they need to be extra careful in the bathroom.

Prevention

There are many things you can do to reduce your risk of falling in your bathroom. The first and simplest thing is to keep it clean. Wipe up splashes of water from your shower as you're drying yourself. Clean up all spills when they happen—don't wait to do it later. Remember that body oils, soaps, shampoos, and conditioners are incredibly slippery. They may even leave a residue after they've been wiped up; you may have to wash the area to get rid of the slip risk completely. Hang up towels and washcloths when you're finished using them; don't leave them on the floor. Because many bathrooms are small, confined spaces, make sure you keep the floor clean of clutter. Don't keep extra supplies on the floor in places where you may trip on them.

As you transition out of a bathtub you face a combination of higher risk conditions: your foot is wet, you are standing on one foot and you're making an unnatural step over a barrier. While you are off balance even the slightest slip will increase your risk for a STF injury. A grab bar located near the edge of your tub will help you maintain your balance if you should slip.

Place a bathmat with a good, non-slip backing just outside your shower or tub. This is the first thing you should walk on when you leave the bathing area; it will dry the bottoms of your feet and provide you will a nonslip transition. Remove any throw rugs that don't have a nonslip backing, as these may bunch or slip and create additional STF hazards. Everyone is different. If you notice that a particular style of bathmat isn't keeping you safe from slips, trips, and falls, replace it with a style that works better for you.

Thom Disch

Not long ago, I bought one of those cushy foam bathroom mats. It looked great and felt good under my feet and it kept me from slipping when I got out of the shower. The problem was that the area in front of my bathtub is also a walking path. So when I walked alongside the bathtub and stepped on the edge of the mat, the plush foam layer caused the mat to rise up on each side of my foot. When I took my next step, I would trip on the raised part of the mat. The first time I did this, it caught me by surprise, but I was able to recover. I thought I must be getting clumsier in my old age. I was also surprised when the same thing happened the next day, and again and again. Luckily, I was able to catch myself and recover each time without falling.

I must have tripped on that bathmat over a dozen times before I realized that the problem wasn't me—it was the bathmat. The bathmat worked fine for absorbing water when I got out of the shower, but it wasn't designed for walkway traffic. When my foot was half on the mat and half off, the foam came up over an inch on each side of my foot, created a tripping hazard. The solution: get a different style of bathmat for this bathroom and move this foam mat to a bathroom that didn't have a walking path alongside the tub.

Tile or polished natural stone are very popular bathroom floors in homes and in hotels. This type of flooring can be very slippery when it is wet. Using a bathmat is a must but don't stop there, the tiles beyond the bathmat are still very slippery. There are transparent vinyl treads that can be applied to these areas. They will make you safer in your bathroom and still maintain the beauty of your tile. (Visit Peopletreads.com for one option).

Of course, the actual shower or bathtub gets slippery, too. Treat the floor of the shower or tub with a nonslip product. There are peel-and-stick bathtub mats or non-slip strips that will help you prevent a fall in the shower or tub. As the population continues to age there has been a trend toward installing barrier-free showers and walk-in tubs in many homes.

The first thing someone will do when they start to slip is reach for something to help them keep their balance. Grab bars, like handrails on steps, are a great way to avoid a fall. Place these inside the shower and on the wall near where you exit. A standard towel rack isn't designed to act as a grab bar, but there are towel racks that will also work as grab bars.

While showers and bathtubs are the number one location for STF injuries in the bathroom, toilets come in second, with over 20 percent of injuries.[83] As we age, we tend to need a little more support and assistance getting around in the bathroom. Grab bars and floor-to-ceiling posts can be installed around the toilet to provide extra support. And raised toilet seats will make sitting down and getting up easier.

---

83   Ibid.

CHAPTER 15

KITCHENS

Like bathrooms, kitchens are high STF areas because they combine water and other spills with slippery flooring. However, kitchens also contain hot stoves and sharp knives, which, in conjunction with a slippery floor, create a different type of danger. Many sources describe the kitchen as a dangerous room, but I was unable to find statistics that looked specifically at in-home kitchens and STF injuries.

Jimmy Fallon

Late night talk show host Jimmy Fallon learned the hard way about slipping and falling in the kitchen. He had to wear a finger splint on his show for several months because he almost lost his finger after falling in his kitchen.[84] He said he tripped and fell on a braided rug that was on the kitchen floor. When he reached out to catch himself, his ring got caught on the counter and almost ripped off his finger. The injury called "ring avulsion" required 6 hours of micro surgery to reattach his finger including using a vein from his foot to replace the crushed vein in his finger. According to Fallon, recovery included ten days in the intensive care

---

84   Frank Pallotta, "Jimmy Fallon Nearly Lost His Finger in Kitchen Accident," *CNN Money*, July 14, 2015, http://money.cnn.com/2015/07/14/media/jimmy-fallon-injury-finger/.

unit and a complete lack of feeling for eight weeks. He was lucky because surgeons were able to reattach his finger; most people with this type of injury will lose their finger.

Fallon commented about tripping on a rug "that my wife loves and I can't wait to burn to the ground." And while he makes a joke about it, the conflict of fashion versus safety is common. We must find a way to maintain a beautiful home and still prioritize avoiding STF injuries.

Prevention

When I was in high school, I worked in a kitchen at a fast food restaurant. One of the mantras we were drilled with was "clean as you go." Apply this rule to your own kitchen. If you spill, stop what you're doing and clean it up right away. Planning to do it later creates a risk you can easily avoid.

Organize: You can also reduce your risk by putting things away when you're not using them. It's a natural reflex to put your hands out to catch yourself and, in the kitchen, it's usually the countertops you try to catch. The problem with countertops is that if there are knives or glass containers on them when you slip, you could end up with a serious cut on your hands. Keep the kitchen clean and organized by putting things away when you're done with them.

Rearrange: Make sure the items you use most often are in low, easily accessible locations.

Use a step stool: If you have to reach for something, use a step stool, not a chair.

Use a safety mat: Placing a rubberized safety mat in front of your kitchen sink not only increases your safety in an area that has an increased slip risk, it's also more comfortable when you're working.

Close drawers and cabinet doors: When we walk, we don't always look down, especially in the kitchen, where we might be distracted by reading a recipe or running to the stove to respond to a timer. If a lower-level drawer is left open, it will catch you right on your shin. Even if you don't fall down, you'll get a very nasty scrape.

Eliminate throw rugs in the kitchen: Using a rug with a non-skid backing is an improvement, but these should never be placed in high-traffic areas.

CHAPTER 16

HALLWAYS

The higher-traffic areas of our homes pose a greater risk simply because we spend more time there. Hallways and walkways are prime locations for slips, trips, and falls but the cause often includes a combination of other factors that have been discussed.

Examples of hallway and walkway conditions that add to STF risk include:

- **Unsecured runners or throw rugs:** These might look great, but if they're not secured, you're increasing your STF risk. If you must have a throw rug or runner you can use a double sided carpet tape to secure the rug to the floor and reduce the risk of the rug slipping out from under your feet but you can still trip over the edge. Or eliminate the risk by getting rid of these altogether.

- **Clutter:** If you see something in a walkway that might cause a slip, trip, or fall, stop what you're doing and fix the problem immediately. Promising to do it later leaves the risk there for other family members and for you the next time you pass this way (if you forget to come back to fix the problem).

- **Poor or inadequate lighting:** Increase the lighting on your walkway. Use brighter lights in your fixtures. And place nightlights along all walkways that may be used at night when the lights are out. You may forget to turn on the lights if you're awoken in the middle of the night and then that dog toy that wasn't there when you went to bed becomes an STF hazard. Accent lighting is a simple and inexpensive way to make your hallway more attractive and make your home safer.

- **Extension cords:** So you want to increase the lighting in one area of a room but there is no electrical outlet there. Running an extension cord is one solution but now you've created another hazard. Secure extension cords with a cord protector to keep them firmly on the floor. Alternatively, you could use tape to secure the cord to the floor, but remember that this is a short-term solution because the tape will wear out or peel up.

- **Slippery flooring:** Some floor surfaces are naturally slippery. Others become slippery because of the products we use to clean them and make them shiny. Floor wax is a great example. What do you do when you clean your floors? Do you wash them and then walk away and leave them to dry? That's fine if there's no one around. But if there's any chance that someone will walk on your wet floor, alert them to the STF risk. Business environments are very good at this because they post a sign, but we often put our loved ones at risk at home because we don't warn them about wet floors.

CHAPTER 17

UNEVEN SIDEWALKS, PATHS, AND WALKWAYS

We expect our pathway to be even. We've been taught to look up or to look people in the eye, which often means we don't notice changes in our path. It doesn't take much variation to create an STF hazard. Most federal, state, and local codes consider a walking surface variation of just one-quarter to three-eighths of an inch to be an STF hazard.[85] To put this in perspective, a quarter of an inch is approximately the height of three stacked nickels. To complicate matters, as we age, we tend to shuffle our feet instead of lifting them. While everyone is at risk for tripping on an uneven walking surface, the risk increases as we age.

---

85   CNA Financial Corporation, "Addressing the Trip and Fall Hazard," *Risk Control Bulletin*, 2010, https://www.cna.com/web/wcm/connect/ca4fb9dc-af90-4835-9223-2fbbd85c93b1/ RC_GL_BUL_addressingthetriphazard_CNA.PDF?MOD=AJPERES.

Kim and Dave

My wife, Kim, runs three to five miles a day. She also works full time, so her runs are limited to weekends and before and after work. As is true for most runners, Kim likes to take different paths to keep her runs interesting. As the seasons change, the amount of daylight changes, so on occasion Kim finds herself running at twilight. Fortunately, we live in a neighborhood where it's safe for her to run in the early evening hours. Unfortunately, like most neighborhoods, the sidewalks are uneven.

One evening last fall, Kim went for her evening run. It was just after daylight saving time ended, so it was darker than usual. She chose her path through the neighborhood, she was near the end of her run when she missed a sudden change in the sidewalk elevation; her toe caught the raised edge and down she went. She got some serious scrapes on her knees and an elbow, and tweaked her hamstring, but thankfully her injuries weren't permanent.

The following week our neighbor, Dave, who is about 90 years old was reading the morning paper and got up to go get the mail. On the pathway to his mailbox he caught his foot on a similar sidewalk problem. In this case when he fell he got a cut on his forehead, broke his nose and ended up with a couple of black eyes. If you live in a neighborhood with sidewalks I'm sure you or one of your neighbors have been walking and engaged in a conversation and stumbled across a similar situation.

With all of these trip hazards an uneven sidewalk was the primary cause, but there were a combination of factors that made those sidewalk situations more dangerous. In Kim's case, poor lighting and fallen leaves combined with Kim's focus on her run and maybe being a little bit tired as she was near the end of her workout resulted in hitting a trip hazard. For Dave, he got up from reading the newspaper and went to get the mail while still wearing his bifocals. The bifocal lens blurred his vision of the sidewalk and as a result he didn't see the trip hazard on his own pathway. And we all have experienced that embarrassing moment when our attention is not on our path and we trip or stumble (remember Chapter 9, "Distracted Walking").

Falls and fall injuries happen when we least expect them. Heightened awareness and preventative measures can help to reduce the risk. Unsafe sidewalks should be replaced. Isolated trip hazards can be repaired by grinding down the raised portion of the sidewalk, mud-jacking up the lower section of the sidewalk, or installing a transition plate on the sidewalk (visit Handiramp.com/product/sidewalk-repair-kit/ for one option). For a temporary warning or a short-term fix, spray paint a bright color on the sidewalk to warn pedestrians of the trip hazard.

We expect hiking paths to be uneven and if you're someone who hikes often, you pretty much know to watch for the unexpected on the trail, including fallen branches and slippery leaves. But one challenge that will catch even experienced hikers is a change in elevation. When a trail is cut on a slope, through the woods, it creates a perfect path for rainwater and a common result is erosion. To minimize the erosion, wood steps are often built into the path. Depending on the slope, you might see one step every ten feet or an entire stairway built into the trail. These steps tend to become very slippery, especially if they're damp from rain or morning dew. Use extreme caution when walking on these wood steps. (You can also install HandiTreads on these stairs, visit Handitreads.com).

Prevention

Be careful. Watch for uneven surfaces. If you're on a path you walk on often, you probably know the STF hazards. But if you're walking somewhere new, keep a closer eye on your path. Also, when you find an STF hazard, contact someone about resolving the problem. If it's a hazard for you, rest assured that you're not the only person who's at risk.

If you find a trip hazard and don't know who to contact, e-mail me at Thom@stoptheslip.com or use the form at Stoptheslip.com/fallhazard/ and someone from our team will reach out to the person or organization responsible and make suggestions about how to fix the problem. You can make a difference by taking an active role in making the world a little safer for everyone.

CHAPTER 18

RAMPS AND OTHER INCLINED WALKWAYS

Passed in 1991, the Americans with Disabilities Act (ADA) requires all public buildings to provide accessible entrances. And according to the US Census Bureau, in 2010, the percentage of adults that had an ambulatory disability, making it difficult to climb stairs, had grown to 12.6 percent.[86] As a result, we've seen an increase in the number of ramps and inclined surfaces being installed in public places as well as in homes across the United States. As our population continues to age, we'll all be seeing more ramps in our future.

Walking on a slope requires you to change your posture. Your center of gravity must be shifted and the angle of your ankle when you step must change to accommodate the slope. Gravity will pull you down that slope so even a gentle slope will create a slip and fall hazard. The slope on most ramps is generally between five and ten degrees (a five-degree slope is the equivalent of one inch of rise for every twelve inches of distance, and a ten-degree slope is two inches of rise for every twelve inches of distance), but that is enough to create an STF hazard. To add to the problem many of these ramps are outside and they're usually open to elements like rain and snow.

---

86   US Department of Commerce, Economics, and Statistics Administration, US Census Bureau, Americans with Disabilities: 2010: 70–131, http://www.census.gov/prod/2012pubs/p70-131.pdf.

Prevention

First, know that a ramp is going to throw off your balance so walk slower and take smaller steps when on a ramp. Second, anytime the ramp is dirty, wet, or icy, it will be more slippery and more dangerous. Make your ramp safer by keeping it clean and free of ice and snow.

Ramps are built out of many materials but the most common are wood, concrete, or metal. Each ramp should be designed to reduce the risk of a STF injury. Wood ramps will absorb water and tend to be slippery when wet; they also become very slippery when covered with snow or ice. Concrete ramps should have proper drainage to prevent water accumulation. Metal ramps should have a non-slip pattern built into their walking surface.

Use salt or another deicer during winter months to help keep your ramp ice free. If your ramp is slippery you can apply or install slip and fall prevention products to make it safer. I also recommend installing a non-slip product on your ramp. (You can install HandiTreads on ramps to provide traction, visit Handitreads.com).

—— SECTION THREE ——

The Business Side of Slips, Trips, and Falls

This section discusses all aspects of business and slips, trips and falls. STF injuries cost the US economy over $150 billion every year. That amount exceeds one percent of the all the goods and services produced by all US businesses.

The work environment creates additional STF risks for employees. This section explores the different types of fall risks that exist and how different work environments impact your STF risk. We will discuss the policies and programs that employers have implemented to reduce STF risk. Data from the Centers for Disease Control and the Bureau of Labor Statistics have shown that implementation of these safety programs will reduce your risk of a STF injury. The results are that even though business environments appear to have more STF risk, the average person is four times more likely to be hurt by a fall injury away from work than when they are on the job.

This section ends by looking at two industries that are focused on slips trips and falls, insurance and personal injury law. We examine three different types of insurance policies—workers' compensation insurance, liability insurance, and personal health insurance—and how each of them is affected by STF injuries. And we look at the legal side of slips, trips, and falls, focusing on personal liability law, the circumstances required for a good lawsuit, and steps you can take to protect yourself and your business from lawsuits.

The Annual Cost of Falls to the US Economy Exceeds $150 Billion

Cost of Unintentional Falls in the USA
Calendar 2010

Result of a Fall	Number Of Incidents	Medical Costs	Lost Wages	Total Cost	Average Cost Per Incident
Deaths	26,009	$622,265,825	$6,657,653,698	$7,279,919,523	$279,900
Hospitalization	992,452	$38,630,888,947	$56,262,339,893	$94,893,228,841	$95,615
Emergency Department Visit	8,043,684	$20,526,698,988	$30,278,638,301	$50,805,337,290	$6,316
Total	9,062,145	$59,779,853,761	$93,198,631,893	$152,978,485,654	$16,881

Data Source: NEISS All Injury Program operated by the Consumer Product Safety Commission (CPSC).
National Center for Injury Prevention and Control, CDC using WISQARS™. Data extracted August 25, 2016.

- This expense only includes lost wages and medical costs, it does not include the cost of pain and suffering, legal or insurance expense.
- This is more than 1% of the total Gross Domestic Product (GDP) of the USA.
- That is the equivalent of the entire median income (before taxes) for three million US families.
- Over 2% of all healthcare spending was spent treating victims of slip, trip and fall injuries.

Factoid #12

At CNA Insurance, Falls Represent Over Half of All General Liability Claims and Costs

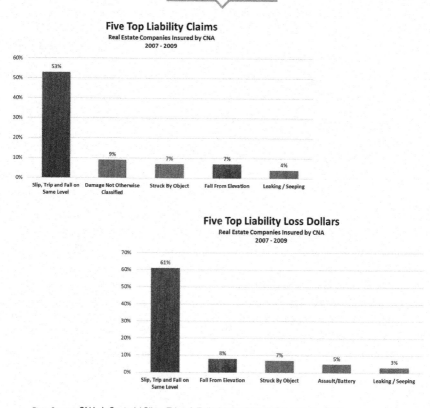

Five Top Liability Claims
Real Estate Companies Insured by CNA
2007 - 2009

Five Top Liability Loss Dollars
Real Estate Companies Insured by CNA
2007 - 2009

Data Source: CNA, InControl / Slips, Trips & Falls for the Real Estate Industry, 2011

Factoid #13

The Cost for Fall Injuries has Grown Much Faster Than Other Workers Compensation Categories

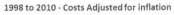

Cost Increase or (Decrease) for the Most Disabling Workplace Injuries

1998 to 2010 - Costs Adjusted for inflation

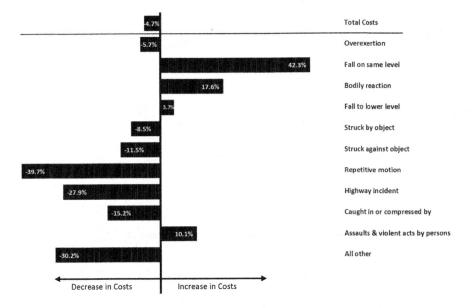

Data Source: Marucci-Wellman, Helen R., et al., "The direct cost burden of 13years of disabling workplace injuries in the U.S. (1998–2010): Findings from the Liberty Mutual Workplace Safety Index," Journal of Safety Research Volume 55, December 2015, Pages 53–62, doi: 10.1016/j.jsr.2015.07.002.

Chart Design: Thom Disch

- Total costs have declined for the most serious workplace injuries.
- Cost for treating the most serious fall injuries has grown by 42%.

Injuries at Work Have Improved

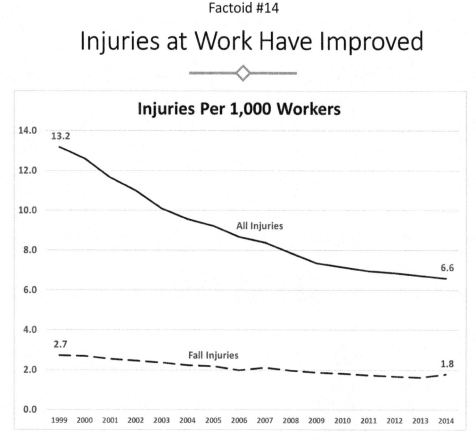

Injuries Per 1,000 Workers

Data Source: U.S. Department of Labor, Bureau of Labor Statistics. Injuries, Illnesses and Fatalities Database. Extracted: Sep 3, 2016

- Overall injuries per 1,000 Workers have declined by 50% during the 15 years between 1999 and 2014.
- Fall injuries have also declined but by a slower pace.
- While workplace fall injuries have declined by 35%, all fall injuries treated in the ER have increased by 9% .

Falls Represent a Growing Problem in Workplace Safety

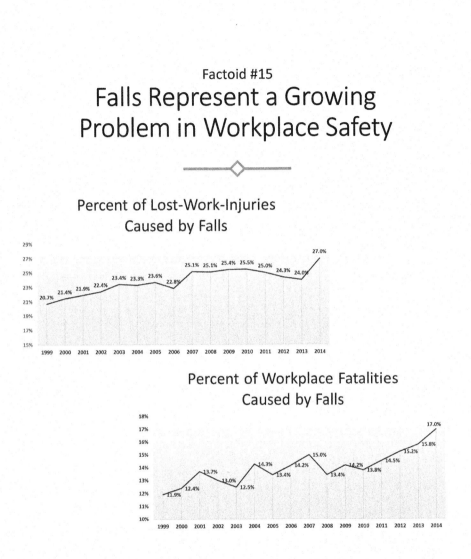

Percent of Lost-Work-Injuries Caused by Falls

Percent of Workplace Fatalities Caused by Falls

- During the past 15 years workplaces have become safer.
- Injuries and deaths from falls have improved but not as much as other causes.
- As a result injuries and fatalities caused by falls as a percent of the total have grown.

CHAPTER 19

THE COST OF SLIPS, TRIPS, AND FALLS

No business section would be complete without a discussion of costs. Since slips, trips, and falls are a complex topic, calculating the related costs is challenging. We're not going to get into the psychological costs, or the costs of suffering, both of which are very real but nearly impossible to value. Legal costs and insurance expense relating to STF are also not included here but are discussed in separate chapters. I want to keep this discussion simple so that we don't get lost in the statistical problems.

The cost of slips, trips, and falls in the United States is large: $153 billion in 2010, as reported by the Centers for Disease Control and Prevention (CDC).[87] Keep in mind that these estimates include only medical costs and lost wages associated with deaths, hospitalizations, and emergency room visits. Those costs were extracted from the WISQARS® system and are displayed in Figure 19.1.

---

87   Centers for Disease Control and Prevention, Data and Statistics (WISQARS): Cost of Injury Reports, https://wisqars.cdc.gov:8443/costT/. Note: The CDC stopped reporting injury costs in 2010, but with healthcare cost inflation and today's higher injury and fatality rates, the actual current cost is much higher.

Cost of Unintentional Falls in the USA
Calendar 2010

Result of a Fall	Number Of Incidents	Medical Costs	Lost Wages	Total Cost	Average Cost Per Incident
Deaths	26,009	$622,265,825	$6,657,653,698	$7,279,919,523	$279,900
Hospitalization	992,452	$38,630,888,947	$56,262,339,893	$94,893,228,841	$95,615
Emergency Department Visit	8,043,684	$20,526,698,988	$30,278,638,301	$50,805,337,290	$6,316
Total	9,062,145	$59,779,853,761	$93,198,631,893	$152,978,485,654	$16,881

Data Source: NEISS All Injury Program operated by the Consumer Product Safety Commission (CPSC). National Center for Injury Prevention and Control, CDC using WISQARS™.

FIGURE 19.1 Cost of unintentional falls in the United States

When we start talking about billions of dollars, my eyes start to glaze over. So let's add some perspective to that number.

In 2010, the cost for falls exceeded 1 percent of the total amount of goods and services produced in the United States for that year. This is a comparison to GDP or gross domestic product, which is the value of all goods and services produced within the US.[88] Putting the cost of slips, trips, and falls into context this means that one out of every one hundred units of *everything* produced in the United States went to pay for the cost of fall injuries. That's one out of every one hundred gallons of gasoline sold, one out of every one hundred homes built, one out of every one hundred hours worked, and, yes, one out of every one hundred McDonald's Big Macs sold in 2010 went to pay for the cost of fall injuries that year.

Hurricane Katrina hit New Orleans in 2005. FEMA called it the "single most catastrophic natural disaster in US history," and estimated the total damage at $108 billion, making it the "costliest hurricane in US history."[89] Keep in mind that Katrina was a one-time event. *Every year,* the cost of STF injuries exceeds the cost of Hurricane Katrina by 40 percent.

---

88   US gross domestic product for 2010 was $14.8 trillion (http://www.bls.gov/ilc/intl_gdp_capita_gdp_hour.htm).

89   CNN Library, "Hurricane Katrina Statistics Fast Facts," http://www.cnn.com/2013/08/23/us/hurricane-katrina-statistics-fast-facts/.

Let's take a moment and focus only on medical costs. The medical costs for treating hospitalization and emergency room visits relating to fall injuries represented over 2 percent of all healthcare spending in 2010.[90] According to the Department of Health and Human Services and the Centers for Medicare and Medicaid Services, total healthcare spending was $2.6 trillion in 2010. Medical expenses for hospitalizations and emergency room visits relating to STF injuries were $60 billion. At first blush, 2 percent of all healthcare spending may not seem like much. But when you realize that all healthcare spending includes *all* health services—from routine doctors' visits to treating everything including cancer and heart attacks and injuries from auto accidents—you realize that 2 percent is consuming a huge amount of our healthcare resources.

One last figure for context: The costs for falls in 2010 exceeded the total amount of money people spent buying new cars in that year. Yes, that includes all Porsches and Mercedes-Benzes and Toyotas and Hondas. If we were to magically reallocate the cost for STF injuries, we could have used that money and bought over seven million brand new Toyota Priuses at an average price of $21,000 each.

---

90   US Department of Health and Human Services, Centers for Medicare and Medicaid Services, "National Health Expenditure Accounts," https://www.cms.gov/Research-Statistics-Data-and-Systems/Statistics-Trends-and-Reports/ NationalHealthExpendData/NationalHealthAccountsHistorical.html.

CHAPTER 20

FALLS AT WORK

In Chapter 3, "Slips, Trips, and Falls: The Inside Story," we talked about how you're less likely to fall *at* work than *away* from work (refer back to Figure 2.7). So, is the workplace environment just naturally safer than other places? There might be some jobs that are safer, a nice desk job perhaps, but when you include all the different work environments, like warehouses and construction sites, and the many different types of jobs, like healthcare workers and restaurant employees, I would have expected that workplaces should be more dangerous. Yet, hour for hour, you're four times more likely to be hurt in an STF accident away from work.

The reason for this has to do with what motivates and drives businesses: money. Businesses have a financial incentive to keep their workers safe. Injured workers reduce productivity, negatively affect morale, generate medical costs, increase insurance rates, and can even result in fines from OSHA. Businesses save money when they train employees and implement procedures that make the workplace safer. They have designated specific individuals to manage the process. These individuals are given authority to make changes and are provided with the financial resources to invest in safer work environments. These individuals *own* fall prevention. They're measured and rewarded based on their success. When you compare this organized, structured environment to your life away from work you can see why you're safer at work. **Who owns STF prevention at your house?**

Even though the workplace does a better job of reducing the risk for slips, trips, and falls than you might in your home, they're still the second most common cause of lost-workday injuries in private industry (just in case you are wondering overexertion is number one).[91] Of course, different businesses have different workplace injury rates. It won't surprise you that employees in an accounting firm have fewer and less severe injuries than workers harvesting timber. It's also true that lumberjacks have more STF injuries than accountants, but we'll examine that in more depth in Chapter 21, "Types of Work Environments."

If we look at workplace injury data, we find that businesses have done a pretty good job of reducing workplace injuries. Since 1999, injuries with days away from work have fallen by 50%, from 13.2 injuries per one thousand workers to 6.6 injuries. Businesses' efforts on STF injury reduction also improved, but the improvement was only 35 percent. You can see the comparison of injury reduction rates in Figure 20.1.[92]

91   National Institute for Occupational Safety and Health, "Preventing Slips, Trips, and Falls in Wholesale and Retail Trade Establishments," *Workplace Solutions*, October 2012, http://www.cdc.gov/niosh/docs/2013-100/pdfs/2013-100.pdf.

92   US Department of Labor, Bureau of Labor Statistics, "Injuries, Illnesses, and Fatalities," http://www.bls.gov/iif/.

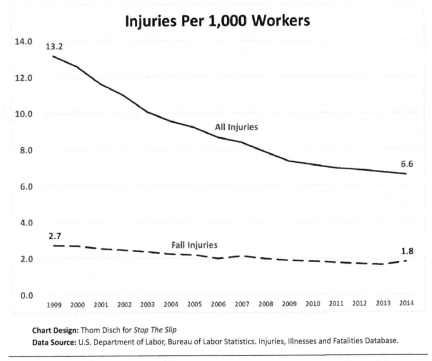

Injuries Per 1,000 Workers

All Injuries

Fall Injuries

Chart Design: Thom Disch for *Stop The Slip*
Data Source: U.S. Department of Labor, Bureau of Labor Statistics. Injuries, Illnesses and Fatalities Database.

FIGURE 20.1 Private labor force injury rates

A 35 percent reduction in the number of STF injuries is very good, especially when the general population has seen a 9 percent increase in STF injuries during a similar time frame. However, the fact that the reduction in STF injuries in the business world hasn't kept up with the overall reductions in injuries means that STF injury reduction should now become a greater priority for businesses. In Figure 20.2 we find that falls, which had represented under 21 percent of all injuries in the workplace in 1999, has grown to 27 percent of all workplace Injuries in 2014.

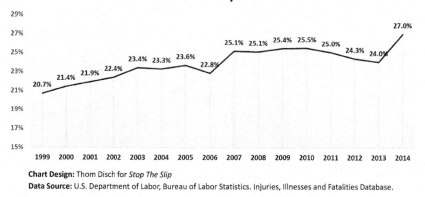

Percent of Lost-Work-Injuries Caused by Falls

Chart Design: Thom Disch for *Stop The Slip*
Data Source: U.S. Department of Labor, Bureau of Labor Statistics. Injuries, Illnesses and Fatalities Database.

FIGURE 20.2 Percentage of Lost-Work-Injuries Caused by Falls

CHAPTER 21

TYPES OF WORK ENVIRONMENTS

Looking across all businesses I was able to identify four types of work environments that differentiate the STF risks for businesses. Examining each of these work environments enables us to identify the factors that cause certain jobs to have more fall injuries than others. Once we understand the differences in each environment, we can create the most effective way to prevent STF injuries in each. The four environments are:

- office and administrative
- production and warehouse
- retail and public
- off-site

Each environment has its own set of risks and challenges. Before we examine each environment let's look at safety in general. One of the first things safety managers are taught is that there are two conditions that lead to injuries: unsafe acts and unsafe conditions. Acts are things people do that result in an injury; people can be trained to do less risky things and ultimately be safer, for example, using a step stool or ladder rather than a chair to extend their reach. Unsafe conditions are environmental in nature. A missing handrail on a stairway is a great example of an unsafe condition. Some conditions are controllable, like maintenance and housekeeping, while others have to be managed as they occur, like the weather.

OSHA tracks the number of STF injuries by industry.[93] When we normalize (number of falls per ten thousand workers), rank, and chart the number of fall injuries per ten thousand employees, we get the breakdown shown in Figure 21.1.

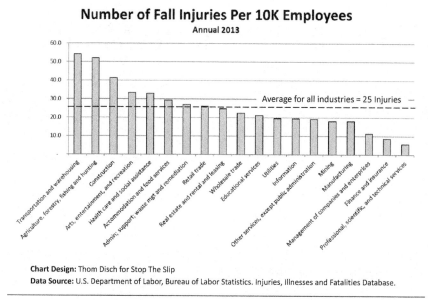

Number of Fall Injuries Per 10K Employees
Annual 2013

Average for all industries = 25 Injuries

Chart Design: Thom Disch for Stop The Slip
Data Source: U.S. Department of Labor, Bureau of Labor Statistics. Injuries, Illnesses and Fatalities Database.

FIGURE 21.1 Number of fall injuries per 10,000 employees, 2013

This information is helpful in analyzing the four business environments. The fact that there are more STF injuries for workers in transportation and warehousing than in professional and technology services isn't surprising. But the fact that the arts, entertainment, and recreation industry has almost twice the fall injury risk of the manufacturing industry isn't quite so obvious. Business environment segmentation may help us to better understand that risk factor.

---

93   US Department of Labor, Bureau of Labor Statistics, "Injuries, Illnesses, and Fatalities," http://www.bls.gov/iif/.

Mark Priest

Complications resulting from an STF head injury resulted in the death of forty-seven-year-old Mark Priest.[94] Priest was a Walt Disney World performer acting in his first show on a new stage when he died from injuries he sustained after slipping on a wet spot. He slipped during a mock sword fight, slamming his head into a wall.

The act was part of Disney's interactive pirate show, in which performers lead park guests through various pirate skills tests. The slip left Priest with a broken vertebra and a head laceration. Priest got up and exited the stage so his bloody injury wouldn't frighten the children in attendance.

Upon arriving at the hospital, Priest was placed in intensive care. Initially he showed improvement and was in high spirits, but he incurred complications from his injuries and died later the same day.

When listing the four environments, I ranked them from safest to most dangerous in terms of STF injury and mortality rates. Let's look at each environment a little more closely.

Office and administrative

This is the safest of the four business environments. This is typically an office environment. The industries that are most comparable are the three safest industries on OSHA's list: management of companies, finance and insurance, and professional, scientific and technical services. This environment requires attention to housekeeping and employee training. The biggest challenges are keeping floors free of clutter, cleaning up spills and wet floors, and training employees to make smart decisions.

Most of the injuries sustained are the result of unsafe acts performed by employees. The best way to reduce STF injuries in this environment is to train

---

94   Barbara Liston, "Mourning Death at the Magic Kingdom," *Time*, August 21, 2009, http://content.time.com/time/nation/article/0,8599,1917776,00.html.

employees on what to watch for and how to maintain a safe workplace. This training should include:

- Using handrails when going up and down stairs
- Using a ladder or stepstool to extend one's reach
- Keeping the floor free from trip hazards, including not leaving items in hallways and not running extension cords across walkways
- Keeping lower file drawers closed when not actively in use

Production and wholesale

This is still a controlled and contained environment. The areas to manage are almost entirely populated by employees and businesses can train employees. More challenging maintenance issues, heavy equipment and tools, and the need to physically move work-in-process and finished product around make this a more dangerous environment. Businesses in the OSHA chart that fall into the production and wholesale environment include manufacturing, mining, and wholesale trade.

The best safety program for these environments will still focus on employee training. Housekeeping, ensuring that work areas free from clutter, and preventing STF hazards should be added to the training program in this environment. Certain job positions will have greater fall risks associated with them; these positions should be identified and extra training targeted to the additional risks.

Retail and public

In the retail and public environment, we add two new factors that will increase STF risk. While the business is still managing our own controlled workspace, that space may have grown, as in the case of an amusement park. We've also added a new population to the environment: the general public.

According to the National Institute for Occupational Safety and Health (NIOSH), a division of the CDC, slips, trips, and falls are the third-highest cause of lost-workday injuries in a retail environment. The primary causes for fall injuries in the environment include: spills on the floor, ice, loose mats/

rugs, poor lighting, boxes/containers obstructing vision, walking surfaces that are in disrepair, and tripping hazards left in a walking path.[95]

The industry fall data does not include injuries to non-employees, but a business that interacts with the public is now faced with a population that they cannot train and, for the most part, cannot control. The most damaging part is that these non-employees (AKA, customers) will change the environment. In the produce isles they drop fruit on the floor or in restaurants they spill their drinks creating additional hazards for other customers and employees alike.

Church Mutual Insurance insures religious institutions of all denominations, including churches, synagogues, and temples. Their operations can include religious-related schools, camps, denominational offices, and senior living facilities. Church Mutual operates in all fifty US states and the District of Columbia. It's the largest insurer of worship centers in the world. Unlike typical retail environments, where workers have storerooms and shelf-stocking responsibilities, workers in religious institutions are exposed to STF risks in an environment very similar to that experienced by their members and guests. And Church Mutual is in a unique position of having to pay claims relating to both employees and the general public (members, volunteers, and guests).

Ed Steele, the risk control manager for Church Mutual, has done some research into STF injuries for employees and for members, visitors, and guests (Figure 21.2). He looked at STF injuries as a percentage of total claims for each of these groups. The comparison revealed that STF claims as a percent of all claims for employees were significantly lower than for members and guests.[96]

---

95 National Institute for Occupational Safety and Health, "Preventing Slips, Trips, and Falls in Wholesale and Retail Trade Establishments," *Workplace Solutions*, October 2012, http://www.cdc. gov/niosh/docs/2013-100/pdfs/2013-100.pdf.

96 Edward Steele, "Managing Your Risks" *Risk Control Manager, Church Mutual Insurance; Risk Reporter for Religious Institutions* 12, no. 4 (Fall 2013), https://www.churchmutual.com/media/riskreporter/pdfs/RRFall2013.pdf.

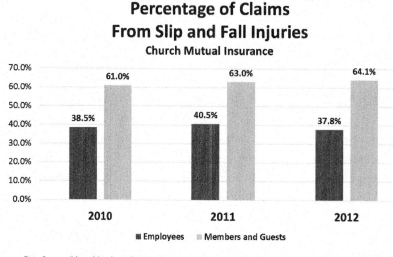

FIGURE 21.2 Percentage of claims from slip and fall injuries

I have two observations about this data. First, while other factors could impact this disparity in claims, a good portion of this disparity is related to an organization's ability to train and manage its employees to avoid STFs. Second, the increase in fall related injury claims for non-employees is huge: 50 percent. In discussing these results with Steele, he stated that the claims numbers at Church Mutual are very similar to the numbers that he saw when he worked for and did similar analyses for both Wausau and Liberty Mutual.

While both employees and customers/visitors have a vested interest in seeing lower fall rates and a safer environment, businesses do not have a convenient way to train and communicate with these non-employees. The untrained actions of these non-employees increase the risks and fall rates for employees. Employees can be trained and penalized for noncompliance with good safety policies. Businesses have no way to train non-employees other than to post polite signs asking for their help. Furthermore, the only way to penalize nonemployees for committing high-risk fall actions is to ask them to leave the premises. And because that action is contrary to the essential reason the business exists, it's implemented only in extreme circumstances.

Businesses that have non-employee interaction have only one reasonable way to address the problem: assigning resources to monitor and clean up after non-employees. This additional monitoring process requires a rigorous schedule for staff to follow so that all areas of the environment are maintained in a safe manor. You never know when a customer will drop a grape on the floor, resulting in an STF hazard for employees or other customers. Employees should be trained to be more observant of accidental fall risks that are created by unknowing customers. We'll discuss legal action in Chapter 23, "Lawsuits and Litigation," but one policy that should be implemented in any business that invites non-employees into its environment on a regular basis is maintaining a written record of safety checks and housekeeping procedures being taken by employees to keep the environment safe for everyone.

Referring back to Figure 21.1, we find that these businesses have fall injury rates above the average rate of twenty-five injuries per ten thousand workers: retail trade; accommodations and food services; healthcare and social services; and arts, entertainment, and recreation.

Off-site

The off-site work environment has the greatest risk for STF injuries. In this environment, the business controls only its employees and their work habits. Examples of business situations include employees being sent onto a construction site to perform work, making deliveries at customer locations, or harvesting crops. The business and its employees have lost total control of the work environment and many times there are other people who aren't under the direction of the business creating additional risks for the employees. In this environment, employees are often asked to do tasks that increase their fall risk and injury rate. The nature of this environment is such that most falls from heights and most fall fatalities occur here. That combination of additional risk factors makes this environment the most dangerous.

The industries with the highest fall injury rates on the OSHA chart all fit into this category: transportation and warehousing;[97] agriculture, forestry, fishing, and hunting; and construction.

It should be noted that most falls from heights occur in this category in conjunction with construction and forestry. Falls from heights are much more dangerous than falls on the same level for obvious reasons. OSHA requires that fall protection be provided at elevations of four feet in general industry workplaces, five feet in shipyards, six feet in the construction industry and eight feet in longshoring operations. In addition, OSHA requires that fall protection be provided when working over dangerous equipment and machinery, regardless of the fall distance.[98]

A summary of the federal rules relating to fall protection from OSHA can be found at https://www.osha.gov/SLTC/fallprotection/standards.html. I should note that in addition to the federal standards issued by OSHA, there are twenty-eight OSHA-approved state plans, operating statewide occupational safety and health programs. State plans are required to have standards and enforcement programs that are at least as effective as OSHA's and may have different or more stringent requirements. To be sure of the rules that apply to your specific location, you'll need to do your own research.

OSHA hasn't ignored fall injuries. Fall protection violations have been the most commonly cited violations issued by OSHA for the past six years (2011-2016).[99] As noted earlier, these violations focus on the risks associated with falls from heights rather than falls on the same level. OSHA has recently approved new rules to address STFs on walking surfaces to become effective January 17, 2017.

---

97 This is a category created by the Bureau of Labor Statistics. If we split transportation and warehousing, we find transportation (off-site) was at 58 STF injuries per 10,000 employees and warehousing was 28 STF injuries per 10,000 employees. Warehousing on its own probably best fits into the production and wholesale environment.

98 US Department of Labor, Occupational Safety and Health Administration, "Fall Protection," https://www.osha.gov/SLTC/fallprotection/.

99 "OSHA's Top 10 Most Cited Violations for 2016," Safety+Health magazine, October 11, 2016, www.safetyandhealthmagazine.com/articles/14927-2016-oshas-top-10-most-cited-violations

CHAPTER 22

INSURANCE

The general intent of insurance is to pool risk. When injuries or accidents happen, the loss is paid from of a pool of funds set aside for this purpose. Insurance allows individuals and businesses to make payments over a period of time and have those funds available to pay for large losses when they occur. Three types of insurance are connected to slips, trips, and falls: workers' compensation insurance, liability insurance, and personal health insurance. While these may overlap, each has its own responsibility and coverage. This chapter is not intended to be a comprehensive discussion of your specific insurance situation, but rather a general overview of the insurance environment. You should discuss your insurance requirements with an expert familiar with your situation and the local rules and regulations that affect you.

Workers' compensation insurance

Workers' compensation insurance, also known as workers' comp, was created to protect employees from the drawn out and costly process of having to sue an employer after a workplace injury or accident. The workers' compensation system was created to provide injured workers and their dependents with timely compensation, regardless of who is at fault for a workplace accident. As part of the legislative compromise that made the employer liable for all work-related injury and disease costs regardless of fault, the employee surrendered the right to sue the employer for injuries. While there are exceptions, workers' comp is typically considered the employee's "exclusive remedy."[100] Workers' comp pays employees for medical costs and lost wages when they're injured relating to their work environment.

Workers' comp is managed on a state-by-state basis. You should consult with a local expert who is familiar with the rules and regulations for your state when making decisions about coverage or claims. Companies may self-insure for workers' comp or they may purchase insurance to mitigate their risk. Depending upon the state, workers' comp may be provided by private insurance companies, by state-run agencies, or by the state directly.[101]

The Bureau of Labor Statistics (BLS) tracks the number of work related injuries, illnesses, and fatalities. Every year they collect this data from businesses using the Survey of Occupational Injuries and Illnesses (SOII) and the Census of Fatal Occupational Injuries (CFOI).[102] The data collected for the Injuries, Illnesses, and Fatalities (IIF) database is fairly comprehensive and contains details that aren't available from the Centers for Disease Control and Prevention (CDC) or private health insurance companies. One limiting factor is that this database relates only to incidents that occur to employees in a job-related situation. Much of the data from the previous two chapters comes from this database.

Although the business world does a better job managing the STF problem than the general public, STFs represent a growing problem for businesses. The severity of an injury can be measured in the IIF database based on the number of days away from work cause by the injury. The Liberty Mutual Research Institute (LMRI) uses this methodology to create its annual Workplace Safety Index (WSI), which ranks the top ten most disabling US workplace injuries for each year based on the direct costs for those injuries. In this report, LMRI

100 Insurance Information Institute, Inc., "Workers Compensation Insurance," http://www.iii.org/publications/insuring-your-business-small-business-owners-guide-to-insurance/specific-coverages/workers-compensation-insurance.

101 Ibid.

102 Dino Drudi, "The Quest For Meaningful And Accurate Occupational Health And Safety Statistics," *Monthly Labor Review* =, December 2015, bls.gov/opub/mlr/2015/article/the-quest-for-meaningful-and-accurate-occupational-health-and-safety-statistics.htm

calculates the cost for all injuries resulting in six or more days off from work, combining incident rates provided by the BLS with data from the National Academy of Social Insurance.[103] While falls on the same level have consistently ranked as the second most disabling injury since 2000, when this report was started, the growth in costs for falls on the same level have shown the most dramatic growth, according to an analysis by members of the Liberty Mutual team.[104] The inflation-adjusted cost for all injuries requiring six or more days away from work actually decreased by almost 5 percent from 1998 to 2010,[105] but the costs for falls on the same level increased over 42 percent. Figure 22.2 shows that no other injury category came close to this level of cost increase.

---

103 Liberty Mutual Research Institute for Safety, Workplace Safety Index, https://www. libertymutualgroup.com/about-lm/research-institute/communications/workplace-safety-index.

104 Marucci-Wellman, Helen R., et al., "The direct cost burden of 13years of disabling workplace injuries in the U.S. (1998–2010): Findings from the Liberty Mutual Workplace Safety Index," *Journal of Safety Research Volume 55*, December 2015, Pages 53–62, doi: 10.1016/j.jsr.2015.07.002.

105 The LMRI, Workplace Safety Index (WSI) reports use data from prior years so that the 2000 WSI actually uses injury data from 1998.

Cost Increase or (Decrease) for the Most Disabling Workplace Injuries
1998 to 2010 - Costs Adjusted for Inflation

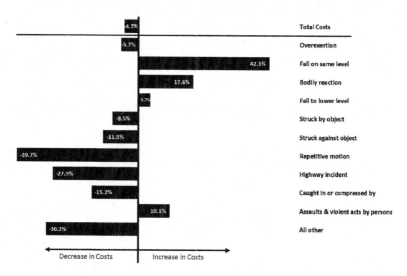

Chart Design: Thom Disch
Data Source: Marucci-Wellman, Helen R., et al., "The direct cost burden of 13years of disabling workplace injuries in the U.S. (1998–2010): Findings from the Liberty Mutual Workplace Safety Index," Journal of Safety Research Volume 55, December 2015, Pages 53–62, doi: 10.1016/j.jsr.2015.07.002.

FIGURE 22.2 Cost Increase or (Decrease) for the Most Disabling Workplace Injuries, 1998–2010

As shown in Figure 22.3, overexertion consistently tops the list of the most costly injuries. Since 2011, STF injuries have been split into three different causes: falls on the same level, falls to a lower level, and slips or trips without falls. All three made it into the top ten. If you were to combine these three into a single STF category, it would move into the number one spot, consuming 29 percent of the costs.

Liberty Mutual Workplace Safety Index
Most Disabling U.S. Workplace Injuries *
Annual Cost - in $ Billion

Injury Data From	2011	2012	2013
Overexertion	$14.20	$15.10	$15.08
Falls on same level	**$8.60**	**$9.19**	**$10.17**
Falls to lower level	**$4.90**	**$5.12**	**$5.40**
Struck by object or equipment	$5.60	$5.30	$5.31
Other exertions or bodily reactions	$4.20	$4.27	$4.15
Roadway incidents involving motorized land vehicle	$2.40	$3.18	$2.96
Slip or trip without fall	**$2.10**	**$2.17**	**$2.35**
Caught in/compressed by equipment or objects	$1.60	$2.10	$1.97
Struck against object or equipment	$1.60	$1.76	$1.85
Repetitive motions involving micro-tasks	$2.00	$1.84	$1.82
Summary of All Slip, Trip and Fall Injuries	**$15.60**	**$16.48**	**$17.92**

* Injuries requiring 6 or more days off from work

Data Source: Liberty Mutual Research Institute for Safety. 2013, 2014, and 2016 Work Place Safety Index. U.S. Bureau of Labor Statistics (BLS), and the National Academy of Social Insurance.

FIGURE 22.3 Liberty Mutual Workplace Safety Index Studies

Liability insurance

If someone slips and falls on property you own or maintain, you may be responsible for costs related to their injury. Liability insurance is designed to protect you from that expense should an accident occur. These costs are the focal point of most liability lawsuits. (See Chapter 23, "Lawsuits and Litigation," for more on that topic.) The costs for fall injuries in these cases are mostly covered by private insurance companies. Most insurance companies do not provide a breakdown of the costs specifically relating to slips, trips, and falls, because they consider that information to be proprietary.

However, CNA does provide that claims data for the real estate clients they insure as a part of their training and education programs, which are designed to increase awareness of key problems and ultimately make people safer.[106] Figure 22.4 shows that for general liability claims, over half (53 percent) of claims are from slips, trips, and falls on the same level. Another 7 percent are attributable to falls from elevation. That means that approximately three out of every five general liability claims are directly attributable to STFs.

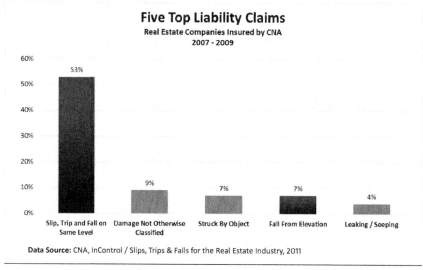

Five Top Liability Claims
Real Estate Companies Insured by CNA
2007 - 2009

Data Source: CNA, InControl / Slips, Trips & Falls for the Real Estate Industry, 2011

FIGURE 22.4 CNA general liability percentage of total claims

And when we look at costs, STFs consume an even greater percentage. Figure 22.5 translates the number of claims into losses incurred or the costs paid by CNA: slips, trips, and falls on the same level consume 61 percent of total liability claims costs for CNA's real estate clients, with an additional 8 percent incurred by falls from elevation.

---

106   CNA, InControl / Slips, Trips & Falls for the Real Estate Industry, 2011,
      https://www.cna.com/web/wcm/connect/570e6da3-d460-4dd7-aaaa-ae931acf7d7e/
      RcBroInControlSTFCommercialRealEstate_CNA.pdf?MOD=AJPERES.

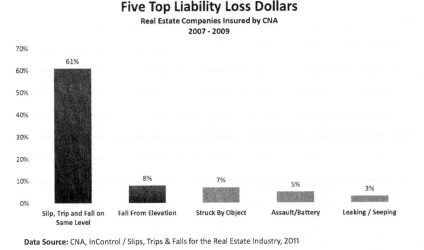

Data Source: CNA, InControl / Slips, Trips & Falls for the Real Estate Industry, 2011

FIGURE 22.5 CNA general liability percent of total claims cost

Personal health insurance

If an injury did not happen at work and wasn't caused by someone's negligence, your personal health insurance will most likely pay for the medical expenses caused by your STF injury. (Personal health insurance also includes Medicare and Medicaid.) Many of these are private companies which are set up differently in each state, so there's no summary data for the costs or size of the total STF problem covered by personal health insurance. You may remember that we looked at data for emergency room visits and admissions to the hospital relating to STF injuries, but the total cost including those STF injuries that didn't require a visit to the emergency room isn't available. If your personal experience is like mine, you go to the emergency room only for the most serious problems. If you can see your own doctor or go to the local walk-in clinic, you do that. If you fall on your front porch, and go to your own doctor, and he diagnoses a sprained ankle, telling you to stay off it for a couple of days, those costs are in addition to the costs previously discussed in this book.

CHAPTER 23

LAWSUITS AND LITIGATION

(This chapter and these examples are not legal advice. The intent is to give you a glimpse at what legal action may entail. Each situation is unique and should be managed accordingly. You should obtain professional legal advice where appropriate.)

Do a Google search for "slip and fall."[107] Google will show you numerous paid ads for lawyers. Okay, no surprise there. In the natural, non-ad section, Google will show you multiple sites where you can find a lawyer and a Wikipedia article on slip and fall. Click on the Wikipedia article and you get a discussion of personal injury claims. The great and mighty Google has concluded that when someone types "slip and fall" into the search box, they must be looking for legal advice. I'm not sure if that's surprising or just really sad statement on the litigious nature of our society. However, it does tell you that slips, trips, and falls represent big business for many attorneys.

Slip-and-fall lawsuits fit into a class of civil cases called "premises liability." These cases come down to an injured person asking for compensation from the company or person that is responsible for the property where the injury happened. There's almost always an insurance company that has insured the management company or property owner. The insurance policy will have a

---

107   This search was performed in the Chicago area on October 7, 2015. Search results may vary based on your location and Google's algorithm.

policy limit and may have some restrictions that will affect the how much and under what situations the property owner will be covered. This is really technical insurance stuff that all property owners will need to work out with their insurance agent. However, as a result of this insurance relationship, most STF lawsuits are negotiated and managed between the injured party, their attorney, and the property owner's insurance company.

How many STF legal actions are there? Quite honestly we don't know. No one tracks this information. I started off by looking at lawsuits. There are two types of courts in the United States: state courts and federal courts. According to the Federal Judicial Center, over 30 million cases are filed in state and federal courts each year.[108] These systems are all managed independently, without any central tracking system. We know that there are a lot of cases filed for STF injuries, but we don't know the true magnitude of that number.

But there's a lot more activity than just cases filed. Not included in these totals is the number of STF cases that are settled before they're even filed. Think about how the system works: Mary slips and falls in the grocery store, breaking her wrist. She calls attorney Bob, whom she found on Google (now that's why Google has so much space devoted to STF lawyers). Attorney Bob calls the store, threatening to file a lawsuit. The store doesn't want to talk to attorney Bob so they refer him to their insurance company.

The insurance company understands the store's liability. They discuss the case and negotiate with attorney Bob. As long as Mary and attorney Bob have a legitimate case and are reasonable in their claims, the insurance company will settle the case without a lawsuit being filed.

As a result, it is impossible to track the number actions and size of the liability from STF injuries. While the insurance companies track all of this data, they don't want to publish it. As you can see from Chapter 22, "Insurance," some insurance companies will reveal portions of the data when it suits their needs for training or marketing purposes.

This process does raise some interesting questions:

---

108   Federal Judicial Center, "Federal Courts and What They Do," 1996, p. 4,
      http://www.fjc.gov/public/pdf.nsf/lookup/FCtsWhat.pdf/$file/FCtsWhat.pdf;

Why do insurance companies settle so many of these claims without going to court?

There are two parts to this answer. The first part is that it's tremendously expensive to go to court. The legal costs to bring or defend a premises liability lawsuit all the way through a trial will total about $50,000 each for both the plaintiff and the defendant.[109] Even after a case is filed, only a small percentage of those cases actually go to trial. Statisticalbrain.com says that only 2 percent of tort lawsuits filed actually go to trial, with the remaining 98 percent settling early. The outcomes of those that do go to trial are pretty much a coin flip, with about 48 percent being won by the plaintiff and 52 percent by the defendant.[110]

The second part deals with the size of the settlement and the likelihood of winning the case. Most of the claims are small relative to the cost of going to court. While the size of the settlement varies by industry, the average settlement in retail environments is about $2,000.[111] Furthermore, the insurance company knows from experience what a reasonable settlement is and which cases it's likely to lose if they go to court. If the settlement amount is reasonable, there's no benefit to the insurance company spending a lot of money to go to trial and then lose.

---

109   Cost of defending from Russell Kendzior, *Falls Aren't Funny* (Lanham, Maryland: Government Institutes, 2010), 31; cost of initiating from Paula Hannaford-Agor and Nicole Waters, "Estimating the Cost of Civil Litigation," *Caseload Highlights* 20, no. 1 (2013), www.courtstatistics.org/-/media/microsites/files/csp/data%20pdf/csph_online2.ashx.

110   Statistic Brain Research Institute, "Civil Lawsuit Statistics," 2016, www.statisticbrain.com/civil-lawsuit-statistics/.

111   J. Hirbyand, "Average Personal Injury Settlements," *The Law Dictionary*, thelawdictionary.org/article/average-personal-injury-settlements/.

Doesn't settling a lot of cases without going to court encourage more claims to be filed?

The short answer is yes. However, insurance companies do not provide any information on how many cases they settle and how many they take to court. That information is highly confidential. Furthermore, the insurance company doesn't give in on every claim. They have a checklist that they use to determine if the claim is legitimate and if the amount being claimed is reasonable. What is on that checklist? That too is confidential and it varies from insurance company to insurance company.

When do insurance companies take a case to court?

Cases will go to court when the insurance company feels that the case may not be legitimate or when the amount being asked for exceeds the amount that they feel is reasonable given the circumstances.

Paula Abdul

Pop star and former *American Idol* judge Paula Abdul had to pay out nearly $1 million to settle an STF claim from an incident that happened in her driveway in 2009. Well, she didn't have to pay it, but her insurance company paid $900,000 and the production company for her reality TV series, *Hey Paula*, paid an additional $100,000 to settle the suit. The size of the settlement combined with the star power of Ms. Abdul landed this story in the headlines. The story behind the settlement can help us avoid similar personal injury lawsuits caused by slips, trips, and falls.

A $1 million settlement is quite unusual; the typical cost for a STF injury is under $25,000.[112] But there were several contributing factors that pushed this settlement so high. Abdul's home in the Hollywood Hills was the set for filming a segment of *Hey Paula* when Jill Kohl, a longtime friend of Ms. Abdul's and a cast member on the show, slipped and fell going down the driveway. Hollywood Hills is where the iconic Hollywood sign is located. Homes in the Hollywood Hills are built on, well, a steep hill. This creates a challenge for builders and architects because the building code mandates a safe slope for driveways and walkways leading up to a home, but the actual "hill" has a much steeper incline. Abdul did not build her home; she bought it from a previous owner (and there may have been a chain of owners since the home was built).

When the architect who designed the home visited the location of the fall, he stated that the existing driveway, brick pavers, and walkway steps weren't a part of his design, which met the building code and had been signed off by the building inspector. At some point after the original construction, the driveway and walkway were changed. A permit for the redesign was never issued by the city and the driveway was never inspected after it was changed. The slope of the driveway at the time of the accident was more than twice as steep as that allowed by the building code. This building code violation laid the blame for the accident squarely on Paula Abdul, the homeowner. Interestingly enough it did not matter if Ms. Abdul

---

112   Average cost exceeds $12,000 from Wausau Insurance; average cost is $22,800 from Don Ostrander, Director Consulting services at the National Safety Council; as reported by Russell Kendzior, *Falls Aren't Funny* (Lanham, Maryland: Government Institutes, 2010): 31, 41.

did the redesign of the driveway or if it was done by a previous owner. In California the responsibility and liability for the property rests solely on the current property owner.

Next, the directors of the segment told all of the cast members to come down the drive rather than the steps, in all likelihood because it created a better visual for filming. At some point Ms. Abdul was caught on tape telling the directors that they had to help her down the driveway because it was so steep. The combination of directing the cast members to go down the driveway instead of using the safer walkway and Abdul's asking for help created what is called "notice." In other words, both the homeowner and the production company were aware that walking down the driveway was unsafe.

At this point the liability for the injury was strongly pointing toward Abdul and the production company. The size of the settlement was directly affected by the extent of Kohl's injuries. When she fell, Kohl severely injured her back. The injury required three spinal fusions, plus rehab, plus time off from work. Add into the equation that Kohl still had chronic back pain even after all the surgeries. The $1 million damages included Kohl's medical bills, which exceeded $400,000, her current and future lost wages, and her attorney's fees, which typically run 30 percent to 40 percent of the settlement.

The insurance company could have forced this case to trial and taken their chances on a verdict that could have totaled several million dollars if it went against Abdul. The legal expenses for taking a case like this to trial would have run about $150,000 for each side. Ultimately, the insurance company decided that to settle the case and avoid the expense of the trial and the risk of a multimillion dollar verdict for the plaintiff.[113]

---

113   The information relating to this case came from multiple sources, including news reports. Robert Clayton of Taylor & Ring, Los Angeles, was helpful in understanding the legal aspects of the case and what both plaintiffs and defendants should do to protect themselves.

Slip, trip, and fall claims (or lawsuits)

How do you know if an STF event can become a legitimate claim or lawsuit? STF lawsuits can be complicated. As you can imagine, they're subjective, meaning that two people may see the same set of facts and come to very different conclusions about who is responsible for the injury and how much damage or expense was incurred. Joel Greenburg, an attorney who has been doing slip, trip, and fall lawsuits for over forty years, provided me with a six-point checklist to determine if there's a claim. You must answer yes to all six items for a claim to be actionable:[114]

1. Was there was a condition on the property which presented an unreasonable risk of harm to people?
2. Was someone injured? (This person becomes the plaintiff.)
3. Was the property owner's negligence the proximate cause of the injury?
4. Did the property owner know or should he or she have known of both the condition and the risk?
5. Was it unreasonable for the property owner to expect that people on the property would see the risk and avoid the danger?
6. Was the property owner negligent in one or more ways?

Most of the legalese has been edited out of this checklist, except for the concept of *proximate cause*. The simplest way to understand proximate cause is to use the "but for" rule. Essentially the proximate cause rule means that an injury would not have occurred *but for* the property owner's negligent action or omission of action.[115] Proximate cause does not establish liability or fault for the injury, but there's no claim if you cannot establish that the property owner was the proximate cause for the injury.

Once a claim passes the six-point test, it moves on to determining the extent of the damages and who is responsible to pay for those damages, or in legalese, liability. The court looks at damages simply as an attempt to put the injured party back in the same physical or financial situation they were in or

---

114   Interview with Joel Greenburg, Chicago, July 2015. Joel H. Greenburg, Ltd.
115   Jeffrey Lehman and Shirelle Phelps, *West's Encyclopedia of American Law,* 2nd ed. (Detroit: Gale, 2005).

would have been in if they hadn't been injured. Punitive damages are damages awarded in excess of actual damages to punish the property owner. Punitive damages are very rare and are awarded in only 5 percent of all civil cases.[116]

State courts and legislatures determine the method for awarding damages from liability claims like STF lawsuits for claims under their jurisdiction. There are two different rules for evaluating blame and awarding damages. The most common rule is comparative negligence. This basically means that someone who may have been partially responsible for their own STF injury may still recover some portion of their damages. Most states and the federal court system have moved to the comparative negligence rule.

At the time of this publication, Alabama, Maryland, North Carolina, Virginia, and Washington, DC, use the contributory negligence rule, where a person will not be able to recover damages if the court determines that the injured person was partially responsible for the accident.[117] Contributory negligence was the original standard in all states but the legal system has been moving toward comparative negligence. (If you're involved in an STF lawsuit, check with a lawyer in your state to be sure which rules apply to you and he or she will help you understand the unique application of those rules to your case.)

Let's walk through a simple example of how comparative negligence would work: the court and the jury are asked to compare the amount of responsibility for causing the injury and then award a portion of the damages based on the responsibility for causing the injury.

Please keep in mind that things are never this simple. Dave slips and falls in a restaurant. He was texting on his phone as he was walking to bathroom when he slipped and fell. His medical bills were his only damages and these were $1,000. If this went to trial, the judge (with an amount this small it would be unlikely that a jury would be involved) would decide if the restaurant was the proximate cause for the fall and then decide how much Dave's

---

116   US Department of Justice, Office of Justice Programs, Bureau of Justice Statistics, Special Report, March 2011, http://www.bjs.gov/content/pub/pdf/pdasc05.pdf.

117   Justia, "Comparative and Contributory Negligence," 2016, www.justia.com/injury/negligence-theory/comparative-contributory-negligence/.

texting contributed to his fall. If the judge decided that the restaurant was the proximate cause for the fall and Dave's texting was 20 percent responsible for his fall, Dave would be awarded $800. The math is simple, but there's no method for determining if texting while walking represents 10 percent or 90 percent of the responsibility for the fall, which is what makes the outcome at trial unpredictable.

Avoiding a lawsuit

In the end, no one wants to be injured in a slip, trip, or fall. The standard is that a property owner must maintain their property in a reasonably safe manner. And visitors must be reasonably cautious when on the property. Insurance companies are very happy to help coach and support the property owner in doing this. They have a vested interest in making sure that the property is safe and free from danger. If you're a property owner, you should use them as a resource.

Here's an example of the action steps for creating a safe environment:

Property owner responsibility

1. Set up a schedule for walking the property. The schedule will be different for different types of operations; a high-traffic fast food restaurant will need to be walked more frequently than low-traffic operations.
2. Create a checklist of what the walker should look for and actions taken if there's a hazard observed.
3. Document who did the evaluation, the date, and the time, and keep this on file.

Creating a safety inspection schedule, and documenting it, will work in your favor if an STF accident should occur. Remember that a property owner doesn't have to eliminate all STF hazards the moment they occur, but they have to show reasonable care in an attempt to maintain a safe environment. I should note that having an inspection schedule can work against you if the schedule isn't maintained (inspections are skipped or forgotten or not documented) as you've established an act of negligence that the injured person can use against you.

Individual responsibility

1. Be aware of your environment; avoid distractions whenever you're walking.

2. Help others; if you notice an STF hazard, fix it if you can. It might be something as simple as moving a hazard out of the way. You can easily move a skateboard from your neighbor's sidewalk to their lawn.

3. If the STF hazard isn't something you can fix, tell someone about the problem so that the property owner is put on notice and can fix it.

4. If you see an STF hazard and don't know who's responsible to get it fixed, submit a video describing the problem at stoptheslip.com/submit-your-video/ and we'll do our best to let the owner know of the problem and help them fix it.

Annette Ritzman

In August 2003, Annette Ritzman, a Williamsburg, Virginia business-woman, slipped on a small puddle and fell outside a convenience store after buying a newspaper. According to the lawsuit and media accounts, a leaky awning caused the puddle.[118]

Ritzman fell forward hitting her chest and chin on the pavement eight inches below the sidewalk. Her head snapped back when her chin hit the ground. She received stiches and was released from the local hospital that same day. She returned to work after a few days of recovery. At work she had a difficult time concentrating and focusing. Then she began to have seizures. Her doctors diagnosed her with post-concussion symptoms. Prior to the fall, Ritzman had been a successful businesswoman. Afterward, she could no longer do her job because she had lost her ability to concentrate and multitask.

A typical STF award is a few thousand dollars. In this case, the jury awarded Ritzman $12.2 million. Her attorney compared Ritzman's problems to those found in a wrongful death case. He explained to the jury that the person her friends and family knew actually died that day, leaving someone else in her place. After her accident, Ritzman lost brain cells and her personality, essentially leaving her a stranger to everyone who knew her. He justified the multimillion dollar award by explaining, "There's no prosthetic brain. You could give her $100 million, it's still not going to replace the brain cells she's lost."

---

118   Seth Freedland, "Woman Awarded $12.2 Million in Slip-and-Fall Case," *Daily Press*, May 2, 2007, http://articles.dailypress.com/2007-05-02/news/ 0705020144_1_wrongful-death-suit-stephen-smith-brain.

SECTION FOUR

Preventing Slips, Trips, and Falls

It all starts with a fall. It is obvious that you can't have a fall injury without a fall. However, we have a false sense of security because in our own personal histories we have survived many falls without serious consequences. Our challenge is that it's nearly impossible to predict which falls will cause injuries and which ones will just be embarrassing. So our mission must be to prevent *all* falls.

Can falls be prevented? Whenever the topic of fall prevention is discussed, I hear one of these two arguments:

- Falls happen to the elderly and are just a part of growing older.
- Falls are caused by things we can't control, like the weather or unseen hazards.

Of course we can't prevent all falls, but there's undeniable evidence that we can reduce STF injuries. My optimism is confirmed by the wide variety of organizations, such as the National Safety Council (NSC), the Mayo Clinic, the Centers for Disease Control and Prevention (CDC), and the World Health Organization (WHO), all of whom have published articles and programs for preventing falls.[119]

Furthermore, we already have proof that injuries and deaths can be reduced with concerted and focused effort. We've reduced the number of motor vehicle deaths by 18 percent while both the number of miles driven and the number of drivers have increased. Furthermore, we've seen that the occurrence of STF injuries and deaths at work are significantly lower than outside of work (see Chapter 2, "Why Slips, Trips, and Falls Aren't Taken Seriously, and Figures 2.8 and 2.9). If we can reduce the risks of an injury while driving and reduce STF risks at work, we can reduce all STF accidents.

We've seen that with a focused effort the number of STF injuries and deaths can be reduced. But the current programs that are focused on reducing

---

119   National Safety Council, http://www.nsc.org/NSCDocuments_Advocacy/Fact%20Sheets/
      Slips-Trips-and-Falls.pdf; Mayo Foundation for Medical Education and Research,
      "Fall Prevention: Simple Tips to Prevent Falls," http://www.mayoclinic.org/healthy-lifestyle/
      healthy-aging/in-depth/fall-prevention/art-20047358; Centers for Disease Control and
      Prevention, "What You Can Do to Prevent Falls," http://www.cdc.gov/
      HomeandRecreationalSafety/pubs/English/brochure_Eng_desktop-a.pdf; World Health
      Organization, "WHO Global Report on Falls Prevention in Older Age,"
      http://www.who.int/ageing/publications/Falls_prevention7March.pdf.

STF injuries for the elderly have not been effective. So I've developed the ALERT System, a five-step program to help reduce the risk of falls and make everyone safer (see Chapter 24, "The ALERT System for Reducing STF Injuries and Deaths").

This section includes checklists for you to use to review your home and business with a focus on how to identify STF risks and avoid injuries.

Falls Kill Seven Times More People Than the Flu

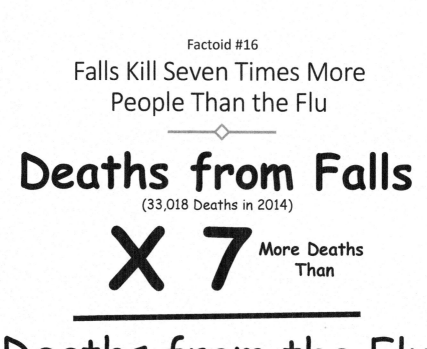

Deaths from Falls
(33,018 Deaths in 2014)

X 7 More Deaths Than

Deaths from the Flu
(4,605 Deaths in 2014)

Data Source: NEISS All Injury Program operated by the Consumer Product Safety Commission (CPSC). National Center for Injury Prevention and Control, CDC using WISQARS™. Data Extracted September 1, 2016.

- We spend $5 billion on flu prevention shots every year. (That does not include the cost of advertising and public service announcements.)
- Over 30,000 people die and 9 million people go to the ER for treatment from fall injuries.
- If we spend $5 billion on fall prevention and awareness every year we could save thousands of lives and reduce the number of ER visits by millions.

Factoid #17

Deaths from motor vehicle traffic has been declining while deaths from falls has been on the rise

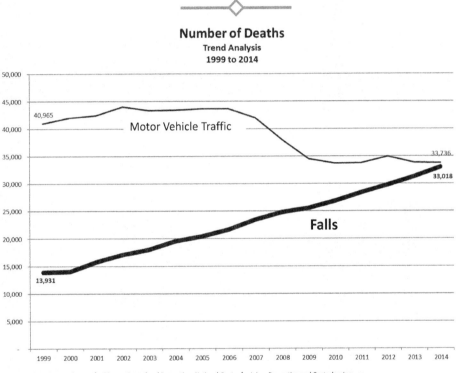

Number of Deaths
Trend Analysis
1999 to 2014

Data Source: Centers for Disease Control and Prevention, National Center for Injury Prevention and Control, using WISQARS™. Data extracted on May 30, 2016

- Deaths from motor vehicle traffic declined by 18% during the last 15 years.
- Deaths from falls has increased by 137% during the last 15 years.
- If these trends continue, deaths from falls will surpass deaths from motor vehicle traffic in 2015.

Factoid #18

Falls Are the Number One Cause of Emergency Room Visits for All Age Groups

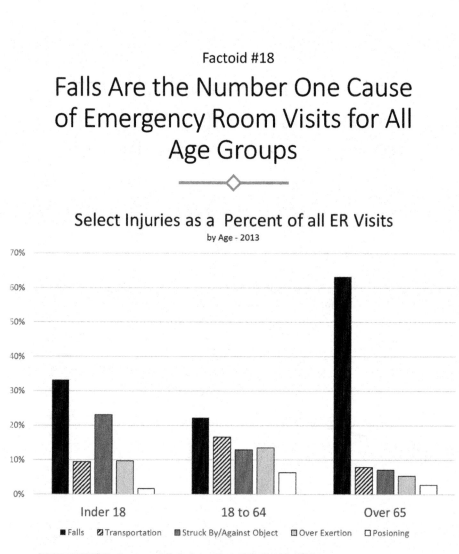

Select Injuries as a Percent of all ER Visits
by Age - 2013

Data Source: NEISS All Injury Program operated by the Consumer Product Safety Commission (CPSC).
National Center for Injury Prevention and Control, CDC using WISQARS™. Data Extracted September 1, 2016.

- Teaching fall prevention to children and young adults will provide a benefit for their entire life.
- Seniors are especially vulnerable to fall injuries.

Factoid #19

The Death Rate from Falls for Seniors Continues to Rise

Deaths caused by Falls
per 100K of Population

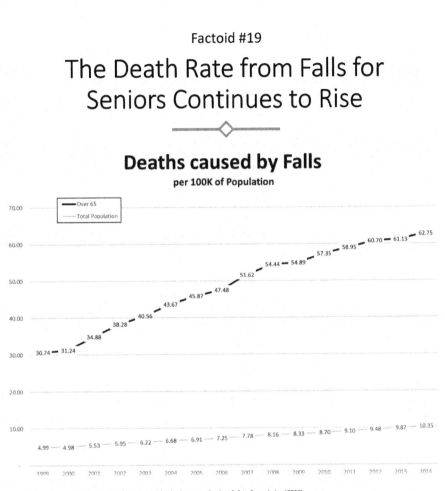

Data Source: NEISS All Injury Program operated by the Consumer Product Safety Commission (CPSC).
National Center for Injury Prevention and Control, CDC using WISQARS™. Extracted September 10, 2016

- For years seniors have been the target of a focused effort to reduce their fall rate.
- The mortality rate from falls for seniors has not improved when compared to the mortality of the total population.

Falls have been the number one cause of emergency room visits in for the past 14 years

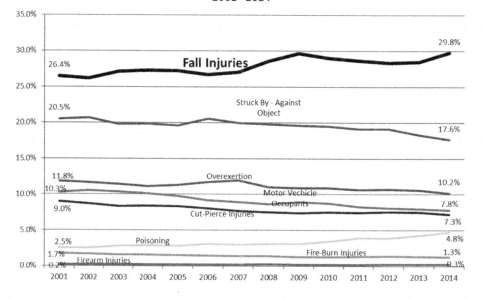

Percent of Emergency Room Visits
By Cause
2001 - 2014

- Fall injuries generate almost 30% of all emergency room visits.
- Falls continue to grow as the leading cause of ER visits.

CHAPTER 24

THE ALERT SYSTEM™ FOR REDUCING FALL INJURIES AND DEATHS

The ALERT System™ for Reducing Fall Injuries and Deaths

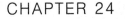

Aware	Learn	Early	React	Train
Awareness is the first and most important step in preventing slip, trip and fall injuries. You should be on alert when you are in higher risk situations. Create a mental slip, trip and fall warning system.	Learn what you can do to prevent a fall accident. Most fall injuries happen in places we know the best: our bathroom, our kitchen, our stairs, etc. This happens because it is our comfort zone, our guard is down and we are not paying attention.	Early awareness, early prevention, and early training will lead to fewer STF injuries for everyone. Fall injuries cause a high percentage of emergency room visits at all ages. Starting the process of avoiding a fall when you are younger will reduce the risk of serious fall injuries when you are older. Start early!	React to what you have learned. If you see a fall hazard, correct that hazard. Do it right when you encounter the risk or problem. Don't count on your memory or your ability to react to a slip or trip risk in the moment.	Train your body and improve your balance. Train your mind to be aware of slip, trip and fall situations. Train your family. Train your friends. Train your co-workers.

© 2016 Thom Disch; Stop the Slip

FIGURE 24.1 The ALERT System™

To successfully reduce STF injuries, we need to approach the problem with a systematic approach. To do this, I've developed a simple, five-step ALERT System designed to significantly reduce all falls (Figure 24.1).[120] We use the acronym: A-L-E-R-T to remind us of the five steps we can take that will reduce the number of falls and fall injuries.

A Awareness is the first and most important step in preventing STF injuries. Be alert when you're in higher-risk situations. Create a mental STF warning system.

L Learn what you can do to prevent a fall accident. Most fall STF injuries happen in the places we know the best: our bathroom, our kitchen, our stairs, and so on. This happens because we're in our comfort zone, our guard is down, and we're not paying attention.

E Early awareness, early prevention, and early training will lead to fewer STF injuries for everyone. Fall injuries cause a high percentage of emergency room visits at all ages. Starting the process of avoiding a fall when you are younger will reduce the risk of serious fall injuries when you are older. Start early!

R React to what you've learned. If you see a STF hazard, correct that it. Do it right when you encounter the risk or problem. Don't count on your memory or your ability to react to a STF problem in the moment.

T Train your body and improve your balance. Train your mind to be aware of STF situations. Train your family. Train your friends. Train your co-workers.

---

120   You can download a printer-friendly color version of this graphic at
stoptheslip.com/book/alertgraphic.

Aware

Awareness is the first and most important step in preventing STF injuries. Your awareness of the problem has already been elevated by reading this book. Now you need to apply that awareness on all areas of your daily journey. Be alert in higher-risk situations. You've read about many common types of fall injuries in the personal stories included here. Add to that by creating a mental STF warning system.

Watch for STF risks. If you slip or trip somewhere, stop what you are doing and take a look at the circumstances related to that slip or trip. Don't assume that you were just clumsy or that your balance and athletic ability will save you the next time. Every year there are nine million emergency room visit examples that prove you wrong.

It's part of our survival instinct to quickly identify dangerous and high-risk situations. Everyone avoids hornet nests and rattlesnakes. If we change our thinking to identify STF risks as dangerous, we then can proactively manage the STF risk to avoid or minimize any potential injury.

It's also your responsibility to spread the word. Pass this same fall-risk awareness onto others so that they can help carry the load. Provide your family, friends, and coworkers with information that helps them understand the risks they face and what actions they can take to be safer. We all need to be part of the solution. This problem is just too big not to share the responsibility.

The Centers for Disease Control and Prevention (CDC) developed a program specifically to help doctors reduce STF injuries for older patients. This program, called Stopping Elderly Accidents, Deaths, and Injuries (STEADI), is a good start.[121] It targets people who are most seriously affected by STF injuries, but it does not address the 75 percent of the fall injuries that occur to the people under 68 years old. The STEADI program needs to be expanded so that people start thinking about STF injuries sooner in life and that means everyone will have more practice avoiding falls by the time they reach the age that will put them at a higher risk of serious injury.

---

121   Centers for Disease Control and Prevention, "STEADI (Stopping Elderly Accidents, Deaths, and Injuries)," http://www.cdc.gov/steadi/index.html.

Learn

Learn what you can do to prevent that STF accident. Learn about your environment. Learn from other people's experiences. Learn from your own experiences. Most STF injuries happen in places we know the best: the bathroom, the kitchen, the stairs, and so on. This happens because we're in our comfort zone, our guard is down, and we're relaxed. We're in them many times a day and we think safe passage is virtually guaranteed because we've walked through them safely thousands of times. And then it happens: we get distracted by the kids, the television, or the phone, and a single misstep creates that fall.

We're aware of the risks, we're aware of the most dangerous situations, we're even aware of why we fall. Now we need to learn what we can do to prevent that STF accident. Learn what products and resources are available to help you reduce fall risks in your life. When you identify a STF risk, make a note—not a mental note but a physical note—and then learn how to fix that risk. If you come across an STF risk situation that you don't know how to fix, e-mail me at Thom@stoptheslip.com and I or a member of my team will respond with a product or a plan that will help you reduce or eliminate that risk.

Change your mindset Slips, trips, and falls happen to all of us. They happen frequently. Most of the time they don't cause us any harm, but the statistics are clear: falls will happen and they can cause tremendous pain and even death (in case you missed it earlier, falls cause nine million emergency room visits, hospitalize over one million people, and result in thirty thousand deaths each year). Learn from every STF incident. That little slip today may result in a big fall tomorrow. Think prevention: When each slip, trip, or fall occurs, what could you have done differently?

STF prevention products There are a variety of products that can help you avoid a fall. Many are readily available at your local hardware store; it's just a matter of installing them. I've tried to avoid blatant self-promotion, but I believe that my company has many of the best products in the marketplace for preventing falls and fall injuries. You should look at our products and decide for yourself if they will help you be safer. You can review many of these products at: Handiramp.com/slip-fall-prevention/. My purpose is to educate you so you can make the most informed decisions about how to reduce your fall risks.

Learn about your personal environment The next two chapters provide you with a checklist and a methodology for you to use to do an STF audit for every room in your home or business. Do a survey of all the locations in your home and workplace that represent fall risks. Learning about high-risk situations now will help you avoid an STF injury later.

Early

Early awareness, early prevention, and early training lead to fewer STF injuries for everyone. We all fall and quite honestly we all fall a lot more that we are willing to admit. We know that falls resulting in emergency room level injuries happen to people of all ages. Over time we discover that when we are younger our bodies are able to rebound from the impact of most falls. As we get older we lose that elasticity and falls result in progressively more severe injuries. This means that nature has provided us with the perfect training ground. If we learn how to avoid falls when we are younger, we will receive that benefit throughout our life.

Most of the existing fall prevention programs are focused on the elderly. These programs have been in place for many years. An effective program or programs would reduce the number of fall injuries and the number of fall deaths among the elderly. Using the CDC's WISQARS database, I charted the number of injuries and deaths per 100,000 population for people over age 65 (Figures 24.2 and 24.3). I was surprised to see that for the elderly, the rate of injury grew by 34 percent from 2001 to 2014 and the rate of deaths more than doubled since 1999.[122] These numbers indicate that the current programs are not effectively serving the elderly.

---

122 Centers for Disease Control and Prevention, National Center for Injury Prevention and Control, Consumer Product Safety Commission, National Electronic Injury Surveillance System—All Injury Program, http://www.cdc.gov/ncipc/wisqars/nonfatal/datasources.htm. Analysis and calculations prepared by Thom Disch.

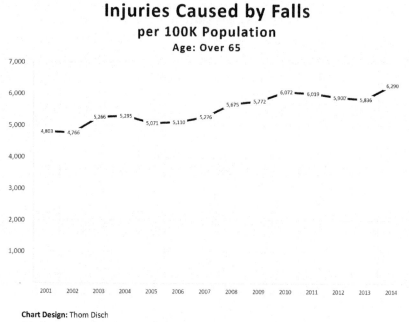

Chart Design: Thom Disch
Data Source: NEISS All Injury Program operated by the Consumer Product Safety Commission (CPSC).
National Center for Injury Prevention and Control, CDC using WISQARS™

FIGURE 24.2 Injuries caused by falls for people over age 65

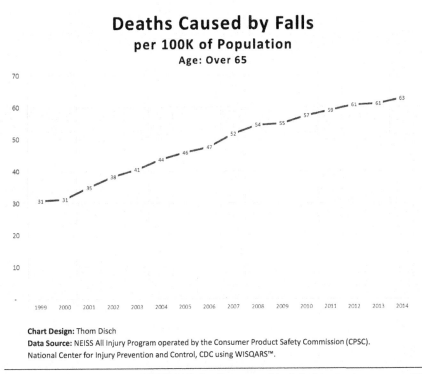

Deaths Caused by Falls
per 100K of Population
Age: Over 65

Chart Design: Thom Disch
Data Source: NEISS All Injury Program operated by the Consumer Product Safety Commission (CPSC).
National Center for Injury Prevention and Control, CDC using WISQARS™.

FIGURE 24.3 Deaths caused by falls for people over age 65

The obvious next question is "Why have our programs and messaging for seniors not been effective at reducing fall injuries and deaths for this group?" I believe there are two reasons: first, that the elderly, who might need the advice, don't consider themselves elderly, so they ignore the message or deflect it, thinking it's for someone else; and second, if they accept the fact that they're elderly and might be at a higher risk for an STF injury, they believe that an STF injury will not happen to them (see the discussion of optimism bias in Chapter 2, "Why Slips, Trips, and Falls Aren't Taken Seriously").

We are faced with a dilemma, the elderly who are at the greatest risk of serious STF injury are not willing to act to protect themselves from these injuries. To solve this problem, we need to re-frame the problem. We need to change the goal and the motivation for seniors. The matriarchs and patriarchs of our families have lead and protected the family for most of their adult life. It should come as no surprise that they are not willing to admit to their vulnerability to a STF injury and they are not motivated to protect themselves from this risk.

The solution: Change the message from "the elderly should help themselves avoid a fall" to "the elderly should help protect all of their family and friends from falls by making fall prevention a priority." This change in motivation is consistent with the perception that most seniors have regarding their role in the family. We have seen that *everyone* is at risk for an STF injury, tasking the most senior members of our society with the responsibility of protecting their family and friends from STF injuries will provide seniors with the knowledge and the tools to help themselves while at the same time train everyone about how to avoid serious STF injuries when they become older.

Yes, we should still emphasize that the elderly are at a greater risk for serious injuries as a result of a fall, but that should be the supporting message, not the primary focus. Additionally, teaching people early, when they're younger, to watch out for STF risks will help them avoid falls when they get older. Asking the elderly to take the lead role in STF prevention because everyone is at risk will help motivate them. They might not do it for themselves, but will they do it to protect their grandchildren? You bet.

React

React to what you've learned. If you see a fall hazard, correct that hazard. Do it right when you encounter the risk or problem. Don't count on your memory or your ability to react to an STF risk in the moment.

Many times, that fall happens in a place that we knew to have high STF potential. Think back during the past month, I'll bet you can think of at least one situation where you were at risk of falling. Now here's the important question: what did you do?

Derek Holland

Derek Holland is a professional athlete. In 2012, he signed a five-year, $28.5 million contract as a starting pitcher for the Texas Rangers. In the 2013 season, he started thirty-three games and pitched 213 innings, with an ERA of 3.42. That's a pretty solid season. At age 27, prior to the start of the 2014 season, he was enjoying a nice night at home with his family, when his dog Wrigley, a boxer, was at the wrong place at the wrong time. Wrigley ran up the stairs and clipped Holland, causing him to fall. His injuries required arthroscopic surgery to repair torn cartilage in his left knee. According to Holland, his athletic abilities were the only thing that saved him from more serious injuries, as he was able to grab the handrail and prevent himself from falling all the way down the stairs.[123] Holland's fall caused him to miss the first half of the 2014 season. He came back after the All-Star break, but his starts dropped to five, with only thirty-seven total innings pitched.

Can we prevent accidents like the one that happened to Derek Holland? In hindsight, Holland's dog could have been better trained, and Holland himself could have been holding on to the handrail before he was bumped, or he could have avoided being on the stairway if he anticipated that his dog was going to be running wildly up or down the stairs. It's hard to anticipate situations like this and it's possible that this was the first and only time Wrigley bounded uncontrollably up the stairs. However, if Holland's household and dog are anything like mine, this wasn't the first time Wrigley bolted by someone on the stairs. The opportunity for prevention in this type of situation comes from recognizing a risky situation that has a high likelihood of being repeated and eventually causing an injury. If we make the effort to recognize potentially dangerous situations when we encounter them we'll be able to correct an STF hazard before it becomes and injury. In this situation, Wrigley's behavior

---

123   Richard Durrett, "Derek Holland Blames Dog for Fall," *ESPN*,
        January 13, 2014, http://espn.go.com/dallas/mlb/story/_/id/10279073/
        texas-rangers-pitcher-derek-holland-clarifies-fall-was-my-dog-wrigley

should have been identified as a problem and then action should have been taken to better train Wrigley, thus reducing the risk.

Train

Life is unpredictable. So is your risk of falling. You can manage your attention level and you can control your environment, but the unexpected is always just around the corner. Having reached this point in the book you have already begun training your mind to be more aware of STF hazards. Training your body will help you respond to the unexpected. Then work to train your friends, family, and coworkers by passing on the word about the universal risks of STF injuries.

Focus your training on creating a level of fitness and improving your balance. However, training programs work only if you actually do them. The best-designed fitness program is useless if you can't motivate yourself to actually participate in it. The benefits from improving your fitness last as long as you're fit. This means participating in a fitness program for a short period of time will help you in the short run, however you'll get the most benefit from including some form of fitness and balance training for the rest of your life. Sound daunting? It doesn't have to be. You can integrate the right program into your current lifestyle. The real challenge is finding the right program for you.

First, always talk with your doctor or healthcare professional before starting any physical fitness plan. But how do you determine the right program or activity for you? I can't help you decide. To be effective you must participate, so it must be something you enjoy. It's also helpful, but not required, to have a partner who participates with you. This will provide that little bit of extra motivation we all need to keep us engaged. When we partner with someone, it puts a little bit of extra pressure on us to participate because we don't want to let our partner down.

Where to start? Not ready for a formal exercise program? That's Okay—any regular physical activity will help reduce your risk of STF injuries.[124] Physical activity strengthens muscles and increases flexibility and endurance. Your balance and the way you walk may improve with exercise, decreasing the chances of a fall. You can also integrate balance training into your everyday activities. For example, try something as simple as standing on one leg while you brush your teeth.

Here are three other activities that will help you with your training and balance:

Walking: Walking is a great place to start. It doesn't require an instructor or a class, although you can sometimes find walking clubs gathering at malls before the stores open for business. It's a safe exercise for most people. You can start walking at any time and you can walk almost anywhere. If you don't exercise at all, it's easy to begin; you already know how to do it. Walking will improve your balance and will contribute toward your overall aerobic activity and physical fitness. Walking also helps build lower-body strength, which is an important part of good balance.

Tai chi: Harvard Medical School claims that tai chi "could be the perfect activity for the rest of your life."[125] Tai chi is a low-impact, slow-motion exercise. You perform a series of motions while breathing deeply and focusing your attention on your bodily sensations. The movements are usually circular and never forced; the muscles are relaxed, rather than tense; the joints aren't fully extended or bent; and connective tissues aren't stretched. Anyone can do tai chi, from athletes, to people confined to wheelchairs, to those recovering from surgery.

The benefits of tai chi may start very quickly. One study compared participating in a three-times-per-week, six-month long tai chi program to a control group that did not participate. The group that learned tai chi significantly

---

124 National Institutes of Health, "Falls and Older Adults," *NIH Senior Health*, http://nihseniorhealth.gov/falls/personalchanges/01.html.

125 Harvard Medical School, "The Health Benefits of Tai Chi," *Harvard Women's Health Watch*, December 4, 2015, http://www.health.harvard.edu/staying-healthy/the-health-benefits-of-tai-chi

decreased their number of falls (by 55 percent) and consequently their fear of falling. Tai chi also improved functional balance and physical performance in those group members that were previously physically inactive.[126]

Learning tai chi requires a leader or trainer and often is part of a structured class. Tia chi classes are often held outside when weather permits. The easiest way to find a tai chi class in your area is to look online. I recommend talking with the instructor and observing a class as a way to begin the process. Your connection to the instructor and the process will determine whether it's right for you.

Yoga: Yoga has different roots and a different process than tai chi, but it seems to produce similar results for improving balance and reducing the risk of a fall, according to a study by the University of Miami School of Medicine.[127] Yoga integrates physical, mental, emotional, and spiritual dimensions to promote health. In addition, yoga can help improve balance and increase confidence in older adults who are at risk for fall-related injuries. The key to successful outcomes is to modify traditional poses in ways that accommodate both physical limitations and fears in the people being trained.[128]

Many YMCAs offer a Moving for Better Balance evidence-based falls prevention program. This program may include Tai Chi and/or Yoga programs. These programs do not require a YMCA membership to participate and they are a great place to start your search for a structured exercise program.

---

126   F. Li, et al., "Tai Chi and Fall Reductions in Older Adults: A Randomized Controlled Trial," *Journals of Gerontology Series A: Biological Sciences and Medical Sciences* 60, no. 2 (2005): 187-194, http://www.ncbi.nlm.nih.gov/pubmed/15814861.

127   Meng Ni, et al., "Comparative Impacts of Tai Chi, Balance Training, and a Specially Designed Yoga Program on Balance in Older Fallers," *Archives of Physical Medicine and Rehabilitation* 95, no. 9 (2014): 1620–1628, http://www.archives-pmr.org/article/S0003-9993(14)00342-6/abstract, doi: 10.1016/j.apmr.2014.04.022.

128   Arlene Schmid, et al., "Yoga Helps Target Falls, Fears in Older Patients," *Lower Extremity Review*, November 2010, http://lermagazine.com/article/yoga-helps-target-falls-fears-in-older-patients.

Practice Makes Perfect

We've all heard, and probably used, the cliché that practice makes perfect. This is the premise behind the Slip Simulator™, a controlled walking path developed by Virginia Tech and Industrial Biodynamics that creates slips, trips, and falls. Participants are fitted with a safety harness that prevents them from actually falling, but when they're on the walkway they're faced with challenging walking situations to create the falling experience without the risk of injury. Participants walk on slippery surfaces, step over barriers, and walk while carrying packages, essentially simulating the STF hazards they face in the real world.

Dr. Thurmon Lockhart, now a professor of biomedical engineering and biological design in the School of Biological Health and Systems Engineering at Arizona State University, founded Industrial Biodynamics while he was studying falls at Virginia Tech. The premise was to address the question: Can we can learn how to avoid slips and falls by actually falling? The methodology combined human motion and injury mechanics with a kinetic learning approach; learn by doing. Using sensors and video, Dr. Lockhart and his team examined the fall risks associated with different activities. These vary based on the tasks being performed by the employees, but the goal is to understand what causes a fall in each situation and how to avoid it. Part of the process is to replicate a high-risk fall situation and then having employees experience that situation. Because people can experience a fall without the risk of injury, they quickly learn which actions and motions are safe and then they can incorporate them into their daily routine. This trial and error method isn't possible in the real world.

Industrial Biodynamics is the company that was formed to bring this technology to businesses to help employees avoid fall injuries on the job. GE Appliances, Westinghouse, Los Alamos National Lab, and General Electric, have used the Slip Simulator and the results have been impressive. According to published results, individuals who took part in the Slip Simulator training experienced a 70 percent reduction in STF accidents.

Even those who just watched others on the simulator experienced a 30 percent reduction.[129]

The training has been primarily applied to workforce and job situations, but now the University of Illinois in Chicago and Professor Clive Pai are conducting a $1 million, five-year study, funded by the National Institute on Aging, to develop a similar treadmill system for the general population, including the elderly. The plan is to train and test thee hundred participants over the next five years.[130] The final results of their study are due in 2018 but they have already they have seen impressive preliminary results reducing falls by 50% in older adults.

The National Council on Aging has many additional training resources available through their evidence based falls prevention program. You can find more information about their initiative and find programs on their website at www.ncoa.org/healthy-aging/falls-prevention/falls-prevention-programs-for-older-adults/.

Training can take many forms. This chapter has focused on the physical aspects of training our bodies. But we should not stop there. We have a societal obligation to pass on this information, to sharing this knowledge with others. We should train our family members, coworkers, and neighbors so they too can *stop the slip*.

129   Alicia Garcia-Lopez, Steven R. Booth, "Statistical Impact of Slip Simulator Training at Los Alamos National Laboratory," http://inbiodyn.com/wp-content/uploads/2016/01/Slip-Sim-Statistical-Significance-Study.pdf.

130   Associated Press, "Tripping seniors on purpose to stop future falls," *USA Today*, August 28, 2014, http://www.usatoday.com/story/news/nation/2014/08/28/tripping-seniors-intentionally/14724251/.

CHAPTER 25

HOME AUDIT CHECKLIST

Continuing in our goal of STF prevention, this chapter is designed to help you observe and correct risks in each area of your home. Look at each area as if you're seeing it for the first time. Go to stoptheslip.com/book/homeaudit and print a checklist for each room in your home. If you don't have access to a computer and a printer, you can use a blank pad of paper to take notes as you review each area:

1. Start at the doorway or just inside the doorway so you can see the entire room. Make a list of all of the pathways you will take when navigating this room or area. This might be a simple single path such as walk down the stairs or could be a list of several different paths that you might walk as you pass through the room.
2. Walk each of the paths you've listed, cleaning up each STF hazard as you walk or making a note to fix bigger problems at a later time.
3. Now turn out the lights. Are you going to have to walk one of these paths when the sun goes down? Where will pets be sleeping or what might be left in one of these paths? Use nightlights to illuminate those paths that will be used when it is dark.

Here are some things to think about as you review each of area in your home.

Bedroom

Make sure the path to the bathroom or out the bedroom door is clear and safe to navigate even after dark. Do not leave clothes or clutter in these pathways. Make a special note of your pet's favorite place to sleep at night. Remember when you wake up at night you will not be fully alert. Better to plan now so that you will be safe later.

Bathroom

Do the shower and bath areas have nonslip treatment? Are there bathmats or shower mats with a good nonslip backing outside each shower area? When you step off the bathmat are you walking onto a nonslip surface? Make sure that towels and dirty clothes are not left on the floor. Keep floors clean and free from soap, shampoo, and conditioners.

Kitchen

Organize your kitchen to keep frequently used items at ground level. If you have to reach up high to bring down items always use a proper stepstool. Keep pathways clear of clutter and clean up spills when they happen. Use a nonslip mat around sink areas. Do not use throw rugs unless they are properly secured using a non-slip product.

Stairways

Keep stairways clean and clear of all clutter. Make sure handrails are solid and secure. Stair treads should be in good repair and treated with a nonslip product. When walking up and down stairs always keep one hand free to hold the handrail. Do not walk up and down stairs in slippery socks. The start of the top of your stairs should be easily identifiable, as people age they may have to mark the start of the stairway with a form of color contrast.

Basement

Keep the basement free from clutter and make sure there are clear safe pathways so you safely navigate around your basement.

Hallway

A hallway is a high traffic area between rooms. The pathway should be clear from clutter and extension cords. All rugs or runners should be secured safely to the floor. Make sure that there are no frayed edges and that all corners stay flatly on the floor.

Living room and family room

Make sure all regularly used pathways are free from clutter and there is enough room to safely walk past furniture. Extension cords should be securely fastened to the baseboards or the floor. Area rugs should be secured to the floor using a nonslip backing that prevents them from slipping. The rug should sit flat on the floor and watch to make sure corners cannot flip up and create a tripping hazard.

Dining room

Your dining room table and chairs should fit comfortably in your dining room. If it's too big, the chair legs will become tripping hazards. Make sure that table runners are safely off the floor. When the dining room is not in use, keep all chairs neatly organized and tucked safely under the table.

Outside

All paths and sidewalks should be level and clean. Keep them free from leaves and shovel them whenever it snows. Use salt or other deicer products whenever the temperature approaches freezing.

Garage

Garage floors are especially dangerous because they get dirty quickly. Your car carries the worst weather conditions inside and even the newest of cars will leave traces of oil under the engine creating a slip hazard. What seems like a large open storage area can become a narrow, trip filled walking path when you park your car. Maintain clean and clear walking paths all around your car so you can safely get from you home to your car and vise versa. You may want to treat your garage floor with a non-slip epoxy coating. Doors with steps leading into your home should have a handrail or grab bar to make getting in and out of your home safer.

Front and back porches

Porch stairs are very dangerous because they are exposed to all of the weather elements. This means rain, and dew, snow and ice, or even the first frost can make the steps very slippery. If your front porch stairs are not exposed to a lot of sunlight you may also have some very slippery mold and mildew growing on them. Often porches are painted and that can make them even more slippery. If your porch is painted, use nonslip paint or install nonslip treads on the stairs. One caution: peal and stick sandpaper tape will not last on stairs that are exposed to a wide variety of weather conditions. The adhesive fails when the changes in temperatures cause the porch surface to expand and contract. Keep the porch and stairs clean and free of dirt and leaves.

CHAPTER 26

BUSINESS AUDIT CHECKLIST

Use the following checklist to reduce the risk of STF injuries in a work environment. This is a basic framework that you can modify to serve the specific needs of your business. Prepare a written action plan for reducing STF risks in each areas of your workplace.

1. Split the business environment into manageable areas. This could be by geographic location, like a single floor or by functional area of responsibility, like shipping, finance, or engineering. Fit the responsibility to what will work best for your business.

2. Assign responsibility for STF prevention for each area to one person, the STF manager. This person will be responsible for monitoring the area and maintaining an STF-free workspace.

3. Next you and the STF manager need to review each area. Start at the entryway to the work area. Position yourself where you can see the entire area. In large work areas you may have to reposition yourself several times to review the entire area. Make a list of all of the pathways that people will take when walking through this area.

4. Rank each path that you've identified for volume of traffic: 1 for high traffic, 2 for medium, and 3 for paths used infrequently by only one or two people. This ranking will help you prioritize which paths are the most important for STF prevention.

5. Walk each of the paths you've listed, make notes of each STF hazard you identify. Fix the problems as you identify them. Track the most frequently occurring problems.

6. Develop a training program to keep STF hazards from re-occurring. This training program should be incorporated into your employee handbook. Putting this program into your handbook reminds everyone how important STF prevention is and will emphasize how important employee safety is to your organization.

7. Develop a program to log all falls into a database. Not all falls with an injury but all falls. What might be a fall without an injury for one person might result in a very serious injury for someone else. This might be difficult as people will be reluctant to report a fall if they think that it will be embarrassing or received negatively. Remember the key to our success is to prevent all falls, not just fall injuries.

8. Set up a scheduled communication program to remind everyone about the importance of fall prevention. This communication plan should include a regular memo about STF successes and failures. List the safest work areas, maybe even tracking of the number of days without a fall for each of your designated areas. You can discuss different fall incidents (without naming names) and what could have been done to prevent that fall the next time.

9. Create a culture of awareness about STF injuries and the problems the cause for society. In a highly visible area, post factoids about fall injuries and the impact they can have on the people in your company. Remember fall injuries that happen outside of work and that happen to loved ones of employees will result in lost work time too. The factoids that are discussed at the beginning of each section of this book are recreated in color and available for you to print and post around your office. You can download them at stoptheslip.com/book/factoids.

Each of the environments discussed in Chapter 21, "Types of Work Environments," has different risk factors. Review the unique challenges for each environment as you write up your safety plan for each area.

CONCLUSION

In reality there is no conclusion. This book is the start of your journey. In Latin, there is a phrase: Semper Vigilans meaning *always watchful* or *always vigilant*, that is how you should approach STF prevention. Safety is an integral part of our lives. We are taught from the moment we begin to walk to look both ways when crossing the street, it is an easy extension to watch for slip, trip and fall risks.

As a part of our ongoing journey we have established the following ways to stay connected:

On the Web: www.stoptheslip.com

This is our central communication tool. You can read our latest findings, find products to fix slip and fall problems, sign up for any of the social media interactions, or request Thom Disch as a speaker at your event or luncheon. We even have a contest for you to suggest a location that needs STF prevention action, or to post your photos of potential STF problems so that we can make suggestions for how to fix the situation. Every once in a while, we'll take your suggestions or photos and offer to fix the problems you've identified for free. (Check out the website for more details on this ongoing project.)

Facebook: www.facebook.com/stoptheslip

Facebook is where friends share information with friends. Here is an opportunity for you to see our most recent updates and to engage in an interactive discussion on our findings, or to share the latest on how to stay safe with your friends and family. We welcome your stories and photos here as well.

Twitter: twitter.com/thomdisch and twitter.com/stoptheslip

We'll send out regular tweets discussing new studies, findings, news articles and celebrity incidents, as well as photos and any news about studies that can help you make better and safer decisions about your home and workplace safety.

Pinterest: www.pinterest.com/stoptheslip/

We'll post a series of STF-related pictures and factoids, along with tips and helpful suggestions about how to reduce the risk of slips, trips, and falls in and around your home.

If you have any questions or comments, please e-mail me at thom@stoptheslip.com and I'll do my best to respond as promptly as possible.

Stay safe!

ABOUT THE AUTHOR

A leading expert and speaker on slip, trip, and fall injuries in the United States, Thom Disch has been compiling statistics and stories related to this healthcare crisis for ten years. He is a serial entrepreneur and owns several companies and nationally known brands, including Handi-Ramp (Handiramp. com), PetSTEP International (Petstep.com), and Industrial Toolz, Inc. (IndustrialToolz.com). He has developed dozens of products for the specific purpose of reducing and preventing slips, trips and falls. These products have won awards for innovation and many of his designs are patented by the US Patent and Trademark Office. He has sold millions of dollars of fall prevention products and solutions to homeowners, businesses and governmental offices. For more information about these slip, trip and fall prevention products visit www.stoptheslip.com/products.

Disch holds a bachelor's degree in economics from Oakland University and a master's degree in management from Northwestern University.

CPSIA information can be obtained
at www.ICGtesting.com
Printed in the USA
LVOW13*2256260418
575091LV00007B/84/P

9 780998 354903